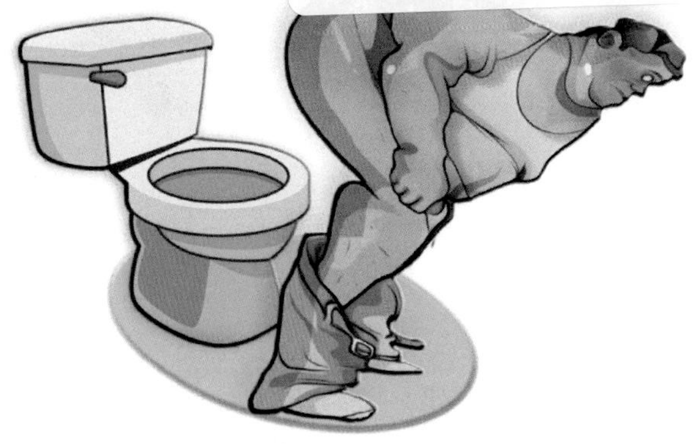

How to wipe your dad's ass

& other things his doctors won't tell you about Alzheimer's.

by

D. Brian Morris

"I don't know what to tell you... I never know what to say to caregivers of an Alzheimer's patient. Just do your best to cope."

~ My dad's doctor when asked how to take care of him ~

Table of Contents

Acknowledgments

I could probably write a second book listing all of the people who helped make this book possible. I only wish I had taken the time to thank the doctors, nurses, paramedics, and fire & rescue personnel who chipped in along the way. The truth is, I don't even remember their names, but I am most certainly grateful for all of their encouragement and help. Inasmuch as I would never be able to find them all and thank them personally beyond what was said during those brief moments we saw them along the way, I would simply ask you, the reader–as a measure of paying it forward—to take a moment from time to time, whenever you encounter one of these unsung heroes, and let them know that you appreciate the fact that they do make a difference. They did for us.

Thank you to my extended family and dearest friends, who pitched in as they could to help us pack and move (to Virginia and to Florida!), or helped with our dogs, or brought food, or sat with dad. To my cousin, Sarah, and her husband Brien, thank you from the bottom of my heart for looking out for Mom and Dad. To my great friend, Don Palmer, his daughter Desiree and her husband Marcus for that god-awful sweltering move from Alabama. *What a nightmare that was! Thank God you were there.*

To my friend, Lee Carr, who helped me with legal language for Chapter 8: thank you so much!

And especially to all of these wonderful proofreaders for volunteering to help me get this thing *finally* wrapped up: Andy and Callie Svenson, Kelly Tarkenton, Shawn Yesner, Lee Carr, Barb Hennessy, Shawn McDermott, and Angie Clark. Without you, this whole thing would have been a collection of typos, misspellings, and grammatical faux pas.

And to all the friends, family, and caregivers I missed... I thank you all. May God's blessing shine upon you always.

Prologue

With my mom holding his right hand, and I his left, my daddy, Lt. Cdr. USN (ret.) Ralph L. Morris, passed away due to Alzheimer's disease on February 17, 2016, at 8:22 p.m. at the Suncoast Hospice Center in Palm Harbor, Florida. He was 74. I had resigned from my job the previous May to help my mom provide fulltime in-home care and moved in with them in November when his condition deteriorated to the point that "24/7" care had become a literal need.

What you are about to read is an earnest attempt to accomplish two things:

1. I'd like to share some truth about what you can expect as a caregiver for a dementia patient; and
2. Hopefully, to prepare you for the day-to-day struggle by giving you some tips from an old man who's been there, done that.

So, as we get started down this path, let us understand at the onset what this book is, and what it isn't.

What it is... This is a book about the ugly underbelly of Alzheimer's written by a guy who actually had to wipe his father's ass on a daily basis. It is the absolute, non-sugar-coated, straight-from-the-hip, no-bullshit assessment of what every Alzheimer's caregiver deals with… Every. Single. Terrible. Long-ass day. It contains unapologetic profanity, raw emotion, sadness and rage all wrapped inside some sort of loving, hopeless care for the one man in this world I loved more than any other with every ounce of my soul. It is a peek into the future for new caregivers with a recently diagnosed loved one. It is a companion to caregivers of patients in the advanced stages (at least you folks will "get it" and perhaps take solace in knowing you are not alone). And maybe in the end it'll even turn out to be a halfway decent "how-to" guide.

What it isn't… This book is not a flowered-up-feel-good-you-can-do-it-yay-rah-rah cheerleading session written by some pansy-ass psycho-babble PhD bullshit artist trying to turn a dollar by telling you everything is going to be okay. Because it isn't. In fact, at the end of the road, your loved one will die from this, just as my dad did, without ever knowing just how hard you had to work to make their last days comfortable, without knowing your sacrifice, and certainly without any expression of gratitude. And you will be left exhausted, heart-broken and, at the same time, mysteriously relieved.

This is not my story. Nor is it my father's. While certain aspects of our lives will, by necessity, be unveiled in this parlance of truth and wisdom, this story is about the struggle of caring for an Alzheimer's patient. It's about the daily grind, the emotions, the mess, the smells, the screaming fits, the tears, the piss-filled diapers, the diarrhea-splattered walls, the sleepless nights, sacrifices, and all of the absolute hopelessness that is this horrid disease we call "Alzheimer's." It will not put you in a good mood. It will not give you a warm fuzzy feeling. And it will not end with "you-can-do-it." Because, who knows? Maybe you can't, but I figure by the end of this book you'll at least have a clue and can plan accordingly.

Oh, and there's one more thing this isn't: the end-all-get-all of Alzheimer's experience and wisdom. This is just one man's point of view among many others. And there's nothing particularly special about me. I have no delusions about that. My situation is not any better or worse than the next. It is what it is.

So . . . Still in? Okay. Grab some ass-wipes and a clean pair of adult diapers, and let's get started.

Chapter 1. Shit.

The first time I had to wipe my dad's ass was in the men's room at Hooters restaurant in Norfolk, VA. I was not prepared. Nor was I remotely aware of how profoundly different my life was going to be after it happened.

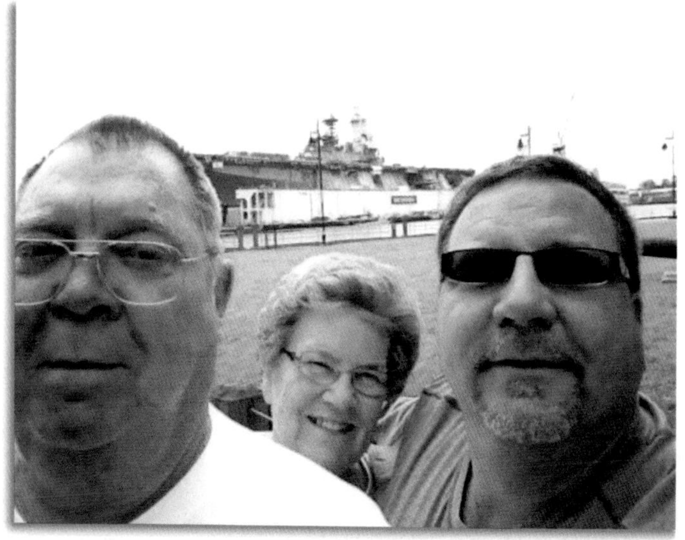

05/10/2014 – Mom, Dad and I wandering around aimlessly in Portsmouth, VA

I was visiting from Florida and had taken my parents out for a day of sightseeing. After meandering through the historic city of Portsmouth and perusing the Port Museum we fell upon the notion that we should have lunch across the river in Norfolk, so we hopped on a water taxi and rode over to the Hooters next to Norfolk's Waterside Marina.

Meals were served, and laughs were had. Then Dad, in what would become a familiar announcement in his booming voice proclaimed, "I gotta go shit."

Well shit, I thought.

Mom told me that he might need some help and asked me to show him to the restroom. *No problem,* I thought. *I'm sure we can find it.* "C'mon, Dad. I'll show you where it is," I gestured, naively thinking that was all that would have been required of me for this little mini-adventure. My ignorance would soon reveal itself in the most absolute terms.

We got to the bathroom, and I showed him the way into the largest of the stalls—the one with the handicapped rails. He settled in to do his business while I took the opportunity to pick an open urinal and relieve myself. Then, while I was washing my hands, I heard him pissing and moaning from within the stall.

"God damn it!... Shit. What the fuck?... Oh, you piece of shit!"

"What's wrong, Dad?" I asked, unknowingly.

"I can't get this piece of shit to work," he said.

"What piece of shit?" I inquired, not having the faintest clue what could possibly be going wrong inside the bathroom stall.

"This... this...", he stammered to find the right word, "shit!"

Timidly, I opened the stall door. He was standing up, pants around his ankles, holding a wad of toilet paper in one hand and unfurling the rest of the roll onto the bathroom floor with the other. He was completely confused and could not figure out how to break off the paper from the roll, let alone what to do with it. I could tell he was as pissed off as he was embarrassed.

"It's okay, Dad. I can help you. Sit back down," I told him.

I picked up all the toilet paper off the floor and discarded the mess. "Do you need me to help you clean up?" I asked, dreading the answer.

"Yes," he sighed. "I think so."

Now the toilet paper at Hooters is of the "John Wayne variety." You know the type... rough and tough, and don't take shit off nobody. So, my first "swipe" set the stage for the rest of the event. The paper disintegrated in my hand,

and I found myself with a handful of shit. Actual shit. Not metaphorical shit. And not just any shit. My dad's shit.

"Shit!" I said out loud and matter-of-factly.

Fortunately, there was a sink close by, and I was able to clean up with relative efficiency. I'm sure the sounds, as well as the conversation emanating from within the stall, were quite entertaining for anyone who wandered through the facilities as we spent the better part of the next 20 minutes cleaning up shit. I'm just glad there was enough of that crappy-ass toilet paper and paper towels to handle the job without having to call the fire department.

We returned to the table where my mom made a joke about him falling in, and I told her what had happened. She was quite unsympathetic. "I have to do it every day," she answered and continued stoically, "did he mess up his shorts?"

Apparently, he was prone to soiling his underwear and pants with some degree of frequency, and I was just learning about the scope of the problem. She went on to tell me that one of his "favorite" things to do at home, when he needed to go to the bathroom, was to pull down his pants the moment he stood up from the recliner in the living room, and start peeing right away as he ventured toward a bathroom 20 feet away, leaving a nice trail of piss along his path, kinda' like breadcrumbs. And God forbid he had a bout of diarrhea! He'd do that, too! So, I learned something that day that I had not expected. He was further down the road than I realized, and we were not prepared. He wasn't *becoming* incontinent, he *was* incontinent.

It was time to change our behavior to accommodate his, and instead of regular Fruit of the Looms, he would need Depends. Due to the fact that his bathroom habits were as unpredictable as they were messy, we would need a few things readily available at all times, and from that moment on we never left the house without a "diaper bag" full of necessities. I've listed them in Figure 1. Packing the Dementia Bag.

Most of the items on the list are self-explanatory. The two that may seem odd at first glance are the KY and the Fleet enema. Which brings me to story two...

The second time I was caught completely off guard in a public place after one of Dad's all-too-familiar "I gotta go shit!" announcements was at a Red Lobster in Clearwater, FL. By this time, I had moved Mom and Dad down to Florida from Virginia, so I could be more hands on with his care. I had no idea how "hands-on" it would be. So, there we were, settling down for a nice lunch at the Red Lobster when—just as the meals arrived in near perfect

Figure 1.

Packing the Dementia Bag

---

1. Several adult diapers
2. Clean flushable wipes
3. Rinse-free perineal wash (in a spray bottle)
4. Disposable latex gloves
5. KY jelly
6. Matches
7. A couple of fleet enemas
8. A complete change of clothes
9. A few plastic garbage bags for soiled clothing

---

timing—he resounded his favorite announcement loudly enough that it turned heads. *Great.*

I ran out to get the diaper bag out of the trunk of the car and walked him into the handicapped stall, helped him onto the pot and waited... and waited... and waited. I watched as he pushed with all his might, his face turning purple as he strained and strained to let loose his pressing troops.

"Well?" I asked impatiently.

"I can't seem to... you know," he struggled to finish his sentence, "do the thing."

He pushed a little more. "Are you done?" I asked, getting more and more pissed off that my lunch was getting colder by the minute.

"I think so," he muttered.

"Okay. Let me wipe your bottom. Assume the position," I barked, ready to eat my meal, now cooling on the table.

He stood up and bent over with his elbows on his knees, and I reached down with a wipe. Then I realized we had a bigger problem. He was impacted. He had a hung turd the size of Gibraltar, half in, half out, solid as marble, and stuck right there! *God damn it.* Any hope of having a warm lunch dissipated instantly.

"Dad, you've got a hung turd! You're going to have to push it out."

He sat down and pressed onward, blue-faced and all, but to no avail. *Well shit. Now what?*

"Okay, Dad, stand up. Assume the position. This is going to be uncomfortable!"

"What are you going to do?" he asked tepidly.

I wrapped my forefinger in a butt-wipe and dug it into the turd, curled it like a fishhook and pulled out as much as I could sweep out.

"Ow, GOD DAMN-IT!!! That hurts!" He screamed.

"I know, Dad, but you're just going to have to suck it up. It's the only way we can get this thing out of your ass. Hold on, here comes the choo-choo!"

He winced and yelped again as I plunged my wipe-wrapped digit into his rectum for the second time. And likewise, on the third. By the fourth probe, he was cold, clammy, pale, and sweating, and I had removed a pretty good amount of the blockage, so I let him sit back down. He flopped back down on the seat with a thump, took a deep breath, and with a mighty heave jettisoned the rest of his oversized payload with a loud pressurized fart and sloshy splash into the commode below him.

He drew a deep breath of relief and softly said, "My asshole burns." He sat there; wet with enough perspiration that you would have thought he had just finished a triathlon in the Sahara. With that, we changed his shirt, cleaned up his bottom and tried to enjoy the rest of our [now, cold] lunch. Suddenly, I wasn't so hungry.

Note to self: add KY jelly, gloves, and Fleet enemas to the diaper bag!

Having told that story, please let me say that while true, it may not have been the wisest thing for me to perform an impacted fecal extraction in a public restroom. Most doctors or nurses will tell you that it should only be done by a professional, which I am not. I only did it out of absolute necessity and would not recommend it. Instead, please be sure to load the KY and enemas in the diaper bag *before* you learn why the hard way. That would only be the first of several times he became impacted, but it was the last time I had to dig it out, thanks to KY and Fleet!

****

Before I leave the subject of "shit," I suppose I should deliver on my promise to describe the best way wipe a grown man's ass. Again, this is from my own experience and may or may not be best for your loved one depending on their mobility, size, and their level of understanding your expectations and directions. At any rate, this is what worked best for my dad:

1. Have him stand up from the commode and lean forward, resting his elbows on his knees (see Figure 2). This will allow easy access to his ass and you won't pinch your hand or arm between him and toilet.

   - Tip: Having him lean sideways on the commode or just lean forward while sitting will NOT work! There's just not enough room between the toilet seat and his butt to get in there and do the thing with any degree of efficiency.

2. Lay an ass-wipe on the open palm of your hand and squirt a liberal amount of the perineal wash on it.

   - Tip: Ensuring that the wipe is good and wet will make the whole process go faster. The wash is pretty cheap, so don't be shy about using it.

3. Starting from his "taint" (the part in the middle that "t'aint asshole and t'aint balls"), wipe towards his anus and use your middle finger to "follow the trench," so to speak. Add a bit more pressure as you cross the orifice to remove as much fecal matter as possible on each pass.

    - Tip: Wiping in the wrong direction will create more of a mess, and you'd then have to clean his balls, too! Always wipe from balls-to-ass, never ass-to-balls! Just sayin'.

Figure 2.

Front-Leaning "Ready Position"

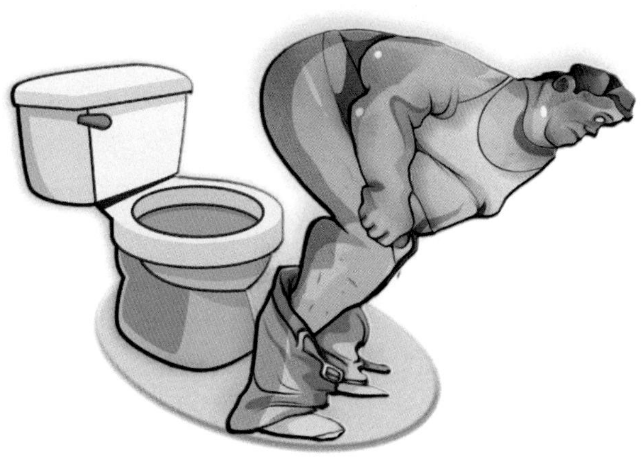

4. Repeat steps 2 and 3 until the valley of the damned is clean—so noted by a resulting clean swipe with no skid marks on it.

    - Tip: Flush often between wipes! My dad could could shit so big he could clog a commode with one good movement and adding too many wipes to that pile of stink could cause a commode to clog so badly that you'd need a team of mining experts to cut through it! Frequent flushing is the key to preventing those fun little nightmares.

5. Finish with a clean wipe without the perineal wash to dry him off a bit before pulling up his shorts.

    - Tip: I also kept matches in the bathrooms at home and in the diaper bag to help eliminate the smell. The free-radical sulfur ions released upon striking a match, along with the available oxygen in the air, bond with the Hydrogen Sulfide (the stinky part of our gaseous anomalies) to form a completely different and odorless gas. It makes the smell go away.

Chapter 2. Hindsight is 20/20.

My dad was one of the smartest men I've ever known. Hell, he's the guy that taught me algebra, trigonometry, calculus, and nuclear equipment qualification. He was a retired naval officer who served for 21 years aboard nuclear submarines. He could calculate complex math in his head, steer large submarines through narrow channels, compute missile trajectories, take a car apart and put it back together without a manual, shoot a bullseye with everything from a .22 caliber pistol to a howitzer, grill steaks to perfection, throw a football with a high degree of precision, hit softballs over centerfield fences, change baby diapers, and tell jokes that would make your ribs bleed; not because he was a good joke-teller, but precisely the opposite. He'd start laughing so hard so long before the punchline that it would take him 15 minutes to tell a 3-minute joke, and we'd all be crying with laughter watching him writhe through it.

And at the end of his life he was reduced to a confused, frightened, incontinent, 300-pound toddler afraid of the dark.

There were many signs. But who knew? I sure as hell didn't.

He was working for me when we first noticed he was "off." He was the CFO for my small but growing ad agency. I had my hands full trying to grow the business, work projects, and manage two locations in Alabama; one in

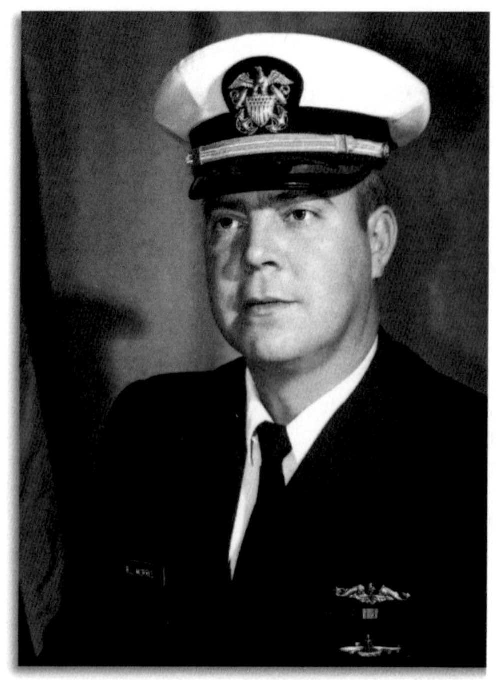

Lt. JG Ralph L. Morris
Vanderbilt Graduation 1971

Cullman and the other in Huntsville. I needed someone I could trust to manage the money. Who else but the guy who taught me how to punch through a differential equation? We had our differences, but I trusted him implicitly. Why wouldn't I?

My first real indicator was a call from my banker. "Hey Brian, this is Tommy Warren. Are you aware that your account is overdrawn?"

"Actually, no I'm not. How much? I'll move money."

"Seven thousand, four hundred dollars."

"What the ff--? Let me call my dad. I'll get right back to you. Don't worry. We'll take care of it today."

Holy shit. $7,400. Are you fucking kidding me?

"Hey," I said to him abruptly, "I just got off the phone with Tommy at the bank. Did you know that we are overdrawn by $7,400?"

"Oh, bullshit!" he said.

"Stop right there. I'm on my way. I'll be there in an hour. When I get there, you'll need to have a better answer than Oh, bullshit!"

Long story short, we moved the money and covered the shortage, but that's not the end of it. It's just one of many examples.

One day he called me at the Cullman office and opened with, "First things first: I'm all right..."

His ominous opening begged the question, "What happened?" Well, he was "fixing" the paper shredder in the Huntsville office and got the brilliant idea to add some lubricant (WD-40, I think) and boom! It blew up in his face, singed his hair, and removed his eyebrows, but he was "all right." Did I mention he graduated from Vanderbilt? Oh, and he was an electrical engineer? He should have known better.

Then there was the time I bought two 12-foot long, 10-inch diameter PVC tubes to attach to the top of our new company van. He was with me when I bought them and knew that I specifically required 12-foot lengths so I could carry photographic backdrops. The backdrops were mounted on 10-foot lengths of 2" PVC pipe and had 10 more inches of mounting hardware added to both ends. He called me the day he mounted them and proudly announced he had "finished." When I got back to the shop, I noticed he had cut four feet off of each tube because they "*looked* too long." He got very angry at me when I reminded him why we needed 12-foot tubes in the first place and had to spend even more money and time to fix his fuck-up.

On another project, we wrapped some graphics on a tour bus for a real estate company. The job was very tedious and expensive. He was given the task of returning the bus to the client 45 miles away, which he gladly did, but not before stopping at the gas station to fill up the tank as a gesture of thanks to the client. The problem? He filled it with regular gasoline. It was a diesel engine.

Then came the day that I finally realized there was something going on beyond a simple inattention to detail. We received payments at both offices, but the accounting was done by my dad in Huntsville. To facilitate ease of record-keeping, I had created a daily report sheet on which any money received at either location was to be duly recorded. One day we received a check for $1,700 in the Cullman office. My mom was the office manager there, and she correctly filled out the daily deposit slip, went to the bank and made the deposit, and then prepared the daily report showing the income. Per procedure, she taped the carbon copy of the deposit slip on the back of the report. She also taped the stub portion of the check to the report, even though that was not required. (Some business checks come with a perforated bottom stub.)

A few days later, I was checking the bank account online when I noticed a $1,700 debit taken out of the account. The note indicated that it was a "miscellaneous" bank fee of some sort. Coincidentally, we had ordered new bank checks at about the same time, and my first thought was that he had ordered $1,700 worth of new checks. I picked up my office phone in Cullman and called my fatherly CFO in Huntsville...

"Hey, did you order those checks?" I asked.

"Yes," He said curtly; he was clearly displeased with the idea that I would question his activities.

"Did they really cost $1,700?" I asked, a bit annoyed.

"Fuck no!" he screamed, now more than a little agitated.

"Well, something's amiss. According to what I'm looking at online, they took out $1,700 for some sort of bank fees. I think they may have mischarged us for the checks. Give them a call and find out."

"God damn it," and [click!] was his abrupt response.

That evening I had dinner with him and my mother at a local restaurant. Of course, I had to ask, "So, what happened about the $1,700?"

"I took care of it," was his stern and abrupt answer.

"That didn't answer my question," I continued.

"I TOOK CARE OF IT!" he yelled with even more angered emphasis.

"Oh, I'm sorry. Let me use language you will understand ... I—the CEO of this company—am asking you, the Vice President and CFO of my company, a direct question. Now, answer the fucking question!" This was phrasing he had used quite frequently over the years as a retired Naval officer, especially when I had worked for him back in the day, so I'm certain he understood that I was not merely going to let it go.

He got up and huffed away from the table; to the men's room, I think.

Then my mother filled me in on what happened. On the day he received the daily report showing the $1,700 deposit, he removed the carbon copy of the deposit slip and discarded it. He then took the stub, filled out a new deposit slip, and re-deposited *THE STUB* it as if it were a check. Why the bank didn't catch that in the first place I'll never know, but they didn't, and they allowed him to make the deposit. The debit was to correct the error, and they didn't know how to code it properly, so it was entered as "miscellaneous" bank fees. My dad was too embarrassed to fess up to his error. I told my mom that she needed to take him to a doctor and get him evaluated. Of course, he refused to go and that ended the discussion.

I'll spare you the details of the daily grind at work. Suffice it to say that dealing with Dad became increasingly more difficult over the two years he worked for me. Mistakes occurred with greater and greater frequency, and his defiance on everything from keeping the books to adherence to the company dress code was unbearable. His inability to keep the books straight meant that I had to do it, which only served to anger both of us all the more. I had no idea why he was being so defiant. I ran the gamut of emotion: rage, disbelief, disgust, and complete depression. It finally came to a head over switching the accounting systems. He insisted on using Excel to keep the books, and he had some convoluted spreadsheet that only he could understand, which meant that if he were to get hit by a bus, we would have been screwed trying to figure it all out, and God forbid if we ever got audited. So, I bought QuickBooks and asked him and our office manager to make the switch. After 6 months of arguing with him over that edict—which he refused to do—I sent him home.

Unless you've been there, I cannot tell you how awful it feels to let someone go. Multiply that feeling a thousand times over when it's a family member. He was clearly unhappy and felt it best to leave and did so with some degree of dignity. At the time, I still had no idea what was at the root of his inability to keep up. The answer was so far off my radar that when we finally found out, it hit me like a sledgehammer to the face, but then it all made sense. I just thought he was being an asshole, because our roles had reversed, and I was no longer his subordinate.

Over the months that followed, my mom complained with increasing frequency that he was doing odd things and making mistakes around the house. Whenever I asked what those were, her answers were always something nebulous, or how he was "just a klutz," and never anything really concrete. He broke this or that or started a project and forgot to finish it. Then one day in the Spring of 2011, she told me about a time they stopped for gas. He went inside to use the bathroom while she pumped the gas. Fifteen minutes later: no Ralph. Twenty minutes gone: still, no Ralph. Finally, after nearly 30 minutes he emerged from the Jet Pep barefoot and wearing nothing but his shorts.

"Good God, Ralph, where are your clothes?" she asked.

"I dunno," he responded with a lost look.

She went inside and found his shirt, glasses, wallet, underwear, socks, and shoes neatly folded in a pile on the men's room floor. That was the straw that broke the camel's back for me. I told her that she had ten minutes to call me back with the name of his doctor and the date and time of his appointment and threatened that if she didn't, I'd would set the appointment for him with a doctor of my choosing and call her back in twenty then drag them both kicking and screaming if I had to. She made the appointment.

And that's how he was diagnosed; nearly two years after I sent him home from work and four to five years after the first onset of noticeable symptoms.

****

Mom and I have often looked back to those pre-diagnosis days and wondered how we missed it for so long. Especially given the fact that his symptoms were so blatantly obvious—hindsight being 20/20. And that's the thing: only in hindsight can you really see how "obvious" the symptoms really are. But when you are living through them, they are hard to pick up for a variety of reasons.

First of all, you're not looking for it and the thought of it actually being dementia just doesn't manifest in your brain; certainly not in the earliest stages of the disease. In our case, there was absolutely zero history of any kind of dementia in our family, and we knew so very little about the symptoms or what to look for. I just thought my dad resented me as a business owner and didn't want to play ball. After all, he was a retired naval commander, and he was not accustomed to being told what to do by a "subordinate" (let alone his own son). He was type A all the way, which only made matters worse whenever we confronted any odd behavior or mistake. The thought process that led me to realize there was something "mentally wrong" was long and complex. In other words, I didn't just "see it" one day and say, "oh, that must be Alzheimer's! Let's go to the doctor!"

For me, it was the check stub incident that made me first think he was losing his mind. It was an absurd mistake, not one of laziness, rebellion, or miscalculation. It wasn't a math error. It was a *mental error*, and knowing my dad, that was a horse of a different color. It was so uncanny and inexplainable that the only conclusion I could draw was that he just "wasn't there" when he made the mistake. Still, he was cognizant enough to argue about it and deny it, and even more resistant to seeing a doctor about it, so his diagnosis would have to wait. It was nearly three years between the check stub deposit and the missing clothes at the gas station.

So, to be clear, there is no "one thing," even in hindsight, that I can point to and say if your loved one is doing this or that, then they definitely have Alzheimer's. It's a sum total of things that are hardest to see in the early stages. From experience, here are some things that Mom and I remember about Dad's behavior that we now realize were dementia-related:

- Failure to finish projects – Dad would start many things around the house but would never finish them.
- Change subjects abruptly in conversation – He would begin sentences talking about one thing and in mid-sentence switch to something else without explanation.
- Confusion when performing simple tasks – It would take my dad hours to do things that he could usually do in a matter of minutes. I once saw him struggle for

over two hours to organize some sockets (by size) in a toolbox; he just stared at them as if they were some kind of mysterious puzzle pieces, then ultimately gave up, and I finished the task for him.

- Getting stuck on words when talking – One of the most common indicators of dementia is the loss of vocabulary. In the beginning Dad would struggle to remember a word or two, but eventually he'd land upon the word or a good synonym to finish his sentences. In the end, he couldn't finish a sentence to save his life. Even a simple, "I'm hungry" was reduced to him pointing at his mouth to indicate he wanted to eat.

- Simple mistakes – Perhaps the biggest indicator was all the mistakes Dad made when fixing things. He used to be a great fix-it guy and jack of all trades. Then... he just wasn't. I've shared a few examples already—the tubes on the van, the paper-shredder, the wrong fuel in the bus, etc. – but there were many others. We made the mistake of ignoring most of them and dismissing them as simple clumsiness and often made jokes of the outcomes and began to refer to him as "Tim the Tool Man" because of his frequent mishaps and similarity to the popular character played by Tim

Allen on the T.V. show *Home Improvement*. It may have been funny then, but it's not so funny anymore.

- Making simple math errors – Like I said, my dad was an electrical engineer; a graduate of the Vanderbilt School of Engineering. A simple math error for him would be like forgetting how to breathe. I remember the day he first looked at the company books. He had this confused look on his face that I thought was him being disappointed with my bookkeeping methods. Even though the books were very well organized and easy to decipher, I attributed his disgust to the notion that they weren't done the way *he* would have done them, which by default would have made them "wrong" in his eyes. I now realize that it wasn't disappointment, it was confusion. He just couldn't follow the math anymore. And rather than admit that—which I understand would have been very embarrassing for him—he covered his confusion with anger directed at me. So, having been scoffed at for "not doing it right," I chalked the incident up to same old dad being impossible to please, told him he could do it however he wanted so long as it was auditable, whiffed off to run my business, and never once considered that he had a problem.

- Misjudging spatial relationships – We moved a lot when Dad was in the Navy, so he had many years of practice packing boxes to move or his bags for travel. His ability to do that, though, deteriorated quickly. I first noticed it when he was working for me and trying to pack boxes for shipping. He went from being a highly logical packer to doing it willy-nilly.
- Diminished driving skills – Wow, this is a big one. Dad was always a pretty aggressive driver and took great pride in getting away with speeding. The rules of the road didn't apply to Ralph Morris. If he were still here, I'm sure he'd tell you why. Nonetheless, aside for his contempt for the speed limit, he was still a fairly good driver until his dementia set in. At first it was mis-judging distances and having to slam on the brakes to make a turn or to avoid rear-ending someone. He'd weave like a new driver struggling to keep the car centered in the lane. He'd miss turns, traffic signs, and lights. He once misjudged the space required for a moving truck he was driving and ran over the front end of a parked car. We finally petitioned the doctor to take away his driver's license on the day he stopped to make a left turn in the middle of a busy four-lane highway with cars barreling at us at 55 - 60 mph. He was too confused to see the entrance to the shopping

center that was right in front of him, and we only narrowly missed being hit.

- Inability to use simple tools – As the dementia progressed, Dad became less and less able to coordinate his hands when using any kind of tools and often tried to compensate by using his fingers; the most obvious sign of this was when he ate. For example, he'd try to use his fingers instead of a fork for foods like spaghetti. Or he would leave huge unshaved patches of his beard when he shaved in the morning. Come to think of it, in the early days, he would often go a few days without shaving, to which I now attribute to his confusion over how to use the razor. In the later days, I had to do that for him, too.
- Inability to keep up with a story line – Often Dad would ask us to repeat things said on the news, or on T.V. shows, or during football games he'd watch. He was a huge Alabama fan and cried when he saw them win the 2012 National Championship because he thought it would be the last one he would see. By the time they won again in 2015, he was so far gone mentally that he could only refer to them as "that red team" and had no idea that they even won the game.

I'm sure there were others, and I could probably fill the whole book if I thought of all of them, but that's not really my purpose here, so I'll leave it with this thought: you *know* your loved one, and everyone is different, so my advice is, if you suspect that he or she is "off," then get them checked sooner than later. There is no known cure for dementia/Alzheimer's (yet), and until there is, I suspect that early diagnosis will go a long way to slowing it down.

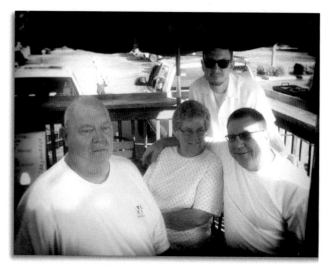

09/24/2015 – Dad, Mom, my son, Scott, and I with Dad at a local restaurant in Dunedin, FL. Notice my dad's expression. He has no clue where he is.

Chapter 3. What's that smell?

From the early days of his disease, Dad became less and less interested in his personal hygiene. There's no other way to put it, he stank! If left unchecked, I'm sure he would have worn the same clothes for days on end. He would have stopped brushing his teeth, shaving, or taking showers, let alone wiping his own ass with any kind of real efficiency. Of course, Mom was absolutely NOT having any of that. After all, she had to sleep in the same bed with the man, and there's only so much stink one woman can take. The occasional fart was bad enough, but this... well, let's just say she was having no part of getting into bed with an old poot whose breath—if bottled by the military—would be classified as an illegal weapon of mass destruction, and who otherwise smelled like shit, piss, and mildewed socks! The trouble is, he never noticed. *This* became one of the long-standing primary battle grounds between the two of them and remained so until he lost the ability to argue with her over the matter; in large part because in the latter days I took over his bathing duties, and he knew better than to argue with me about it.

His resistance to bathing, brushing his teeth, and shaving stemmed (I think) from the fact that he had lost the ability to think through and perform those things on his own. He was embarrassed not by his odor, but by his growing disability to perform the simplest of tasks that most of us take for granted. And so it went...

He normally showered in the morning right after he woke up. In the early stages, his bathing only required some basic supervision and reminders ("Wash your hair... Don't forget to use soap... Clean your tallywacker!" Stuff like that). As the disease progressed, however, supervision became less and less of a "verbal command" job and more and more of a "hands-on" ordeal. It would take Mom over an hour to get him up, get him cleaned, get him dressed, get him fed, and get him to his recliner planted in front of a T.V., which is the only place on earth he wanted to be if not in bed. By then, she'd be completely exhausted and that was at the *beginning* of each day. I always wondered why it took her so long. I found out after I moved in. He fought her. I think there was still some part of his brain that remembered this was his wife—the person he was supposed to protect and take care of, not the other way around. I'm speculating of course, but knowing my dad's nature and ego, I'm certain this was not acceptable to him on any level, and he fought it to the very end *[with her].*

From our side of the fence (mine and Mom's, that is), there was a natural aversion to the whole thing. Seriously, who wants to give their dad a bath? I certainly wasn't thrilled with it, and at some level I resented having to do it. I mean, nothing says *I love you, Dad*, like reaching down to his undercarriage and polishing his big harries, am I right? Bottom line is that neither Mom nor I really wanted to do the thing. It just wasn't right ...or fair ...or fun. It just fucking sucked.

Little did I know that all of my anger and growing bitterness over the matter would one day fall away, because, of all things, an infected dick. One day he sat down to pee and complained like a little boy to my mom that his pee-pee hurt. She took a closer look and found that the head of his penis was bright red, swollen, and covered in some kind of flaky rash. She nearly fainted and gasped at the sight! After getting over the shock of it, she immediately screamed for her resident nurse (me) to come in and assess the situation to see if we needed to go see the doctor.

"Look at his pecker!" She popped, "I think he has some kind of disease!"

Now before I go any further, let me just say that examining my dad's John Henry has *never* been one of my personal "goals," and the thought of doing it at this particular juncture was certainly not something I wanted.

"Do *what?*" I retorted in disbelief.

"Look at your dad's pecker and see if we need to go to the doctor," she repeated, confirming my horror.

And there the three of us were: Mom and I standing above Dad in this tiny bathroom (barely big enough for the commode and certainly not meant for a party of three), her scared shitless, me perplexed and dreading the next few minutes like a man fixing to get gang-raped in prison, and Dad still sitting on the throne with a hurt look in his eyes holding fast to his fire-infected penis!

Fuck my life! "Okay, Dad, stand up... let's have a look."

He stood. I knelt. (Shut up!) and there it was. A red, swollen, infected grown man's dick with a... is that a... well, fuck me...

"He has a diaper rash," I said. I may be his son, but I'm also a father, and I have changed a diaper or two in my day. I've seen diaper rashes before, and this one was a beast.

In an instant, I realized that the reason he had a burning billy-stick was because we (Mom and I) had failed to ensure he was properly clean down there. *He* couldn't do it alone. He needed help. My help. And suddenly all of my disdain, resentment, anger, and hatred for the task of giving him baths melted away. He was like a child. A toddler. I had truly lost my dad.

I cried all the way to the drug store to buy some diaper cream. When I got home, I took him back to the bathroom and had him drop trou. I dropped to my knees, and rubbed a big glob of goo on his dick. The relief was instant. "That feels better," he sighed.

"I know, Dad," I returned. *I know...* And from that point on, I made sure he was thoroughly washed head to toe—ass crack, coconuts, jimmy-johnson and all—every time I bathed him. He never had another diaper rash.

****

Bathing your dementia patient will be a daily ordeal, especially if they fight it. Let's face it, not many of us would really want someone else cleaning and probing our naked bodies. It has to be embarrassing and uncomfortable, so the first step is to have a bit of empathy for their vulnerable predicament. If it sucks for you, too damn bad. Suck it up, buttercup, because I can guarantee you that they would rather be doing it themselves than have you or some stranger cleaning them in the most intimate way. Nonetheless, it has to be done, and here are some tips to make the whole disgusting process a bit more efficient:

- If at all possible, use a walk-in shower; preferably one without sliding doors, because they will try to step barefoot on the rails, which abruptly ends with a slip and fall. Eventually, I physically had to reach down, grab my dad by each ankle one at a time, and guide each foot over the ridge. If your bathroom has a walk-in with doors on rails, my advice would be to remove the doors and rails to facilitate ease of entry and egress. The doors are just going to get in the way, so you might as well just remove them temporarily, so you won't have to work around them. And I can already hear your objections... but, but it'll get the whole bathroom wet. Well... let me clue you in my brothers and sisters, you're gonna get wet. The bathroom's gonna get wet. That's all part of the program. So, yeah... get over it.

- If you don't have a walk-in and are forced to use a bathtub, there are some seats you can buy that will facilitate the transition into the tub. I never had to buy one of those, so I can't tell you with any experience how efficient they may be. I do know they exist, and you can get them at a medical supply place or find them online.
- Install an extended shower head with a long hose; the longer the better. I can't emphasize this one enough. As the disease progresses, they will become less and less able to follow your instructions to move and turn. Having a long hose will ensure that you can get water where it needs to be without having them move. In the latter days (before we had a hospice caretaker coming three times a week), I would have Dad stand in the stall with his back to me with his hands against the far wall of the shower (like he was being frisked by the police), and I could bathe his whole body head to toe in about 5 minutes. You'll get better and faster with experience.
- Get a shower seat for them to sit on (Dad couldn't stand for long before he would get tired and needed to sit). In mid-stages, Dad could kind of wash himself,

but it would take forever, so having a sturdy seat in the shower was essential to his limited autonomy. Plus, it ensured he was relatively still during the process which reduced the probability of slips and falls.

- Don't leave them alone! If I wasn't there to provide guidance, he'd just play with the soap and barely rub it on his belly, and he would completely skip over his genitals, which is what caused the aforementioned rash. You have to remember, they no longer have any concept of personal hygiene or, for that matter, the purpose of soap! It's on you—whether you like or not—to ensure their cleanliness. Not doing so can literally cause them much pain.
- Use tearless shampoos, because they will definitely forget to close their eyes, and it will break your heart when it happens. One time in particular, I was washing Dad's hair (what little of it he had), and the soap trickled into his eyes. His immediate response was to reach up and rub his eyes with the hand in which he held a bar of soap! Needless to say, it was several hours before his eyes stopped burning. Like I said... liquid soap, washing gloves, tearless shampoos. Check!
- Use a washing glove! Those things are great.
- Use liquid soap.

- Use an electric razor to shave your men. At first, I used the same old standard razors he always used. I'd put the cream on his face and shave him. It's odd now to recall those days... to the very end, even though he couldn't remember my name, he knew exactly how to contort his face to facilitate a clean shave. I think about that every single day when I look in the mirror to shave my own... but I digress (sorry). At some point, I switched over to an electric razor, and that made shaving him much more efficient with far less mess and clean-up time.
- Dry and dress them quickly. My dad's metabolism was always out of whack, and he always felt cold. The last thing you need on top of dealing with an Alzheimer's patient is to have to deal with a *sick* Alzheimer's patient!

Chapter 4. Shut the fuck up and go to sleep!

"Get the fuck out of here!" he screamed at the top of his lungs. "I'll kill you, mother fucker! Get away from me, God damn it! Go away!"

"Hey, Dad... you want some ice cream?" I responded softly. "Here's a bowl just for you. It's a good batch this time. It's fresh. I just made it," I finished in a calm, slow voice.

Dad instantly settled down and got very quiet. His night terror had come to an abrupt stop at the simple suggestion of a cold bowl of homemade ice cream. He rolled slightly and, with a deep satisfied breath, fell back into a deep sleep.

If you think dealing with an Alzheimer's patient is challenging when they are awake, brother, let me tell ya'... dealing with them at night is just absolutely, friggin' splendid! Welcome to the wonderland of night terrors, sleepwalks, and the joy of "Sundowner's Syndrome."

With Dad, there was a definite progression in his evening behavior from bad to worse to unbearable. In the beginning, it was just a bunch of bad dreams; by the end, it was sleepless nights, wandering around with his pants down, pissing [or shitting] down the hall, getting up, lying

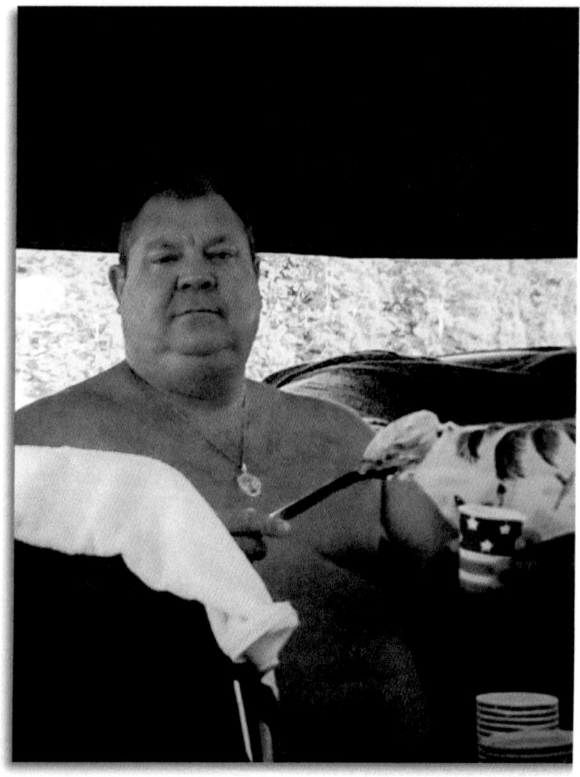

Summer 2002 – Dad and his favorite homemade vanilla ice cream on Smith Lake, Arley, Alabama

down, getting up again. It was relentless, and I can't begin to count the number of nights I stayed up all night long with him for the sole purpose of keeping him out of his bedroom, so Mom could get some much-needed sleep.

Night terrors were the first stage of noticeable sleep disorders with my dad. They occurred nightly and caused much consternation with my mom, who bore the brunt of his violent outbursts which often included kicking and swinging. In 54 years of marriage, my dad never once hit or threatened my mom with any sort of violence. But it became very apparent, very quickly, that these night terrors were becoming a threat to her physical safety. We asked every doctor we saw what could be done about them, and their only answers were sleep medications. That's all well and good, but then you have to deal with a 300-pound, drugged-out zombie, which is no fun either.

During Dad's nightly bouts with his internal demons, Mom—angered by her inability to sleep—would yell at him to shut up and go back to sleep, and I could hear the commotion from three rooms away. I realized, though, that in order to confront these battles, it would require a different strategy.

Now, this is what I know to be true about such situations: *logic doesn't matter.* What I mean by that is this: you cannot argue logically with an illogical mind. First of all, Dad was *dreaming.* Secondly, he was dreaming in a *demented state.* And Lastly, he was not *thinking.* That meant that I would never succeed with an assertive logical command like, "shut up and go back to sleep!" Instead I had to *interrupt* the dream pattern. And that is exactly what I did with the ice cream. The suggestion of a freshly made bowl of homemade ice cream took my dad's mind out of the terror and into a pleasing, comfortable place; probably a warm summer day on the boat dock on Smith Lake where we often made a variety of the cool, creamy treat. Who knows, but one thing is for certain: he loved the stuff, and that simple suggestion brought his mind out of the fight and into his "happy place." He calmed right down and went back to sleep.

****

My suggestions for dealing with night terrors of a dementia patient are these:

1. Don't yell at them. They're not in any sort of logical place, and their bad dreams are likely filled with all manner of scary things that we'll never understand.

Yelling at them doesn't help matters; in fact, it only exacerbates the problem.

2. Remain calm. Their mind is out of control, so you must be in control. Speak as quietly, softly and calmly as possible. The goal is to get them to calm down. You'll never get them to do that by being mad, excited, loud, or curt.

3. Break the pattern. Think of something calm and happy that they like; for example, ice cream, fishing, puppies, kittens, baseball, sleeping babies, hobbies (building models, knitting, crocheting, painting, sculpting, photography, etc.), whatever invokes some sense of calm, happy thoughts in your loved one. As I'm typing this, I'm wondering what a gently suggested, "shhh, the baby is sleeping. Here, you hold him," might do to calm someone down. *ANYTHING* happy and quiet to get them out of the fight and into a relaxed state. Oh, and by the way... you might want to make a list of different things. The ice cream didn't always work, and over time I used several different subliminal suggestions.

****

And so it went... Every night was new challenge, but eventually the night terrors did seem to subside, only to be replaced with Sundowner's Syndrome. Looking back, I'm not so sure which was worse. At least with the bad dreams, he'd eventually fall asleep, but with Sundowner's, not so much.

Sundowner's Syndrome is marked by two things: the incessant desire to go to bed when the sun goes down and the incessant desire to get right back up!

This was the source of some very long, frustrating nights. Every day, we'd get Dad up, get him showered, clothed, fed, and into his favorite chair where he'd spend most of the day watching T.V. or dozing. Often, we would take him out in an effort to prevent him from sleeping the day away, but his attitude toward such trips devolved as his Alzheimer's progressed, even to the point that going out became an exercise in futility as he just wanted to stay home and sleep. Of course, the doctor's only solution was to prescribe more medication to try to make him sleep through the night, which never worked as planned. It only made Dad harder to deal with, because the meds only served to decrease his lucidity.

A typical evening would go something like this:

As the sun went down and the daylight dimmed, Dad would wake up from his full day of dozing and announce, "It's time to go to bed!" Never mind that it's as early as 5:30 p.m. during standard time or only as late as 8:30 p.m. during daylight saving time. Normal bedtimes in our house would be between 11:00 and midnight depending on the day of the week and how early we may have to wake up the next day.

"It's not time to go to bed," we would respond, "Sit tight and watch T.V. with us for a while."

"No, God damn it! I want to go to bed now!" he would scream back.

Now, I know what you're thinkin'... *why not just put him to bed, for crying out loud?* Well, let me tell ya' why... It's because, he wouldn't go to bed and stay there! Every night we would endure his pissing and moaning about going to bed. Sometimes we would keep him up until we actually went to bed, but most of the time, we'd go ahead and tuck him in around 9:00 p.m., which meant I'd have to get up with him, take him to the bathroom—more often than not I'd have to administer a fleet enema so he could shit—wipe his ass, get him dressed down for bed, brush his teeth, guide him to the bedroom, pull the covers down, put on his CPAP mask, lay him down, pull the covers up, stroke his forehead, tell him goodnight, and turn out the light as I walked out.

...and then right about the time I got back to the living room, we could hear him getting up—usually denoted by the loud crash of his CPAP machine hitting the floor because he got up without taking off the mask. So, back to the bedroom I'd go to put him back down. This cycle would repeat a few times until I'd usually bring him back to the living room to watch T.V. for a "few more minutes." That would last about 15-20 minutes (on a good night) before he barked that he wanted to go back to bed. And back and forth we'd go until Mom finally decided to go to bed with him.

Then we'd take him to the bedroom, lay him down, and she would crawl into bed next to him. I'd usually stay up a while longer to see if he'd actually go to sleep. Sometimes he would, but never before a few iterations of being yelled at by my mom to "lay down and go to sleep!", who—in her own futile efforts to sleep—became increasingly agitated at him for his continued restlessness. On many occasions, more and more frequently as his disease progressed, I would get him out of bed and bring him to the living room, then stay up with him all night so Mom could sleep. In the later days of his sickness, I would average about two to four hours of sporadic sleep on any given day.

Mom and I were always exhausted having to deal with his evening adventures. On some nights, he would fall asleep for a few hours before getting up and wandering around the house. I usually slept with my bedroom door closed, and many a night he'd come to my room, crack the door open and simply say, "Hey." It usually meant he had to go to the bathroom and needed help. It's odd now to think back about those nights and realize that no matter how bad it got, even after he forgot my name and only referred to me as "that boy", he always knew where to find me for help. So I'd get up, take him to the bathroom, change his diaper, and tuck him back into bed; if there was still any sleep-time left, that is. Otherwise, I'd just get up, plant him in his chair, and start making breakfast.

My parent's room had floor-to-ceiling, sliding glass, mirrored closet doors adjacent to my dad's side of the bed, so when he woke up, the first thing he'd see was his own reflection. On the more comical nights, you could hear him talking to his reflection in the mirror...

"Hey... how ya' doin' over there on your side?" he'd ask his reflection. Sometimes he'd even stand up and have full-blown conversations with his newfound friend. On one of those occasions, right after the familiar clatter of his CPAP hitting the floor, I was walking back to the room and heard him say, "shhh... here they come. They're gonna make us be quiet." As if he was a child preparing to be scolded.

"What's going on, Dad?" I asked him. This time with Mom following right behind me into the room.

"Nothin'," he said with a guilty child's look on his face as if he had just broken a favorite statue, or a lamp or something.

"Who ya' talkin to?" I inquired.

"That guy," he said pointing to his reflection in the mirror.

"That guy?" I pointed and responded back, "Is he your new friend?"

"Yeah," he said, sheepishly.

Just for fun, I pointed to my own reflection, and asked, "Well, what about that guy? Is he your friend, too?"

"No!" he said matter-of-factly, "that guy's an asshole!"

Mom and I burst into laughter so hard that we nearly pissed our pants. We still joke about it to this day. This was our life every night for the last 6 or 7 months of his life. In fact, when hospice admitted him into their facility, we were under the impression that it was to "regulate his sleeping for a while" to see if they could get him back on track. We were optimistic. I think they knew better.

****

Okay, so what do you do about Sundowner's Syndrome? Well... the short answer is deal with it the best you can. Now having said that, and knowing full well it's a shitty answer, all I can say is no one person can deal with an Alzheimer's patient alone. It takes a team. Mom and I worked as best we could as a pair of caregivers, and we were always exhausted. It stressed us to our limits. Hindsight being 20/20, here are some things I wish had been different:

- On the few occasions that a doctor ordered it, we would have a day nurse, a physical therapist, or an orderly to come and occupy Dad's time for a bit, so we could enjoy some respite from the daily grind. The trouble was that this type of doctor-ordered therapy was only temporary and would only last for a few weeks at a time per the conditions of Medicare/Tri-Care. We did hire some help to come in two or three times a week to babysit while Mom and I went shopping (or just got out of the house), but even that ultimately became too expensive. I would highly recommend hiring a caregiver, if at all possible, as often as your budget will allow, even if it is just once a week or every other. I cannot overstress the value to your own mental health and wellbeing to get away for a few hours to simply take a breath and regroup.

- Work in shifts—preferably with at least three people. If we had a third person to help, I think we would have been much less tired and irritable. As a two-person team, Mom and I managed, but it was still very difficult, and we were always exhausted.

- Try to stay calm. This is tougher than you think when you are sleep deprived. One time I was so tired that I bit Dad's head off. When it happened, I hadn't slept more than an hour a night in nearly three days. I could hear myself screaming at him as if it were an out-of-body experience, and I was a third person watching it instead of participating. I can barely recall what I said, but I know it hurt his feelings very much. Even though he had forgotten it by the next day, it bothers me still. So, by all means, try your best to remain calm, even when they lash out. The calmer you are, and the better you are able to speak in warm, relaxing tones, the more likely they will calm down.

- Remember too, that medicines have a profound effect on them. Dad was sometimes prone to delusions that were hard to decipher and deal with. This was especially true at night after his nightly meds. You must be cognizant that everything you are experiencing, no matter how ridiculous, is a thousand times worse for them, because they have lost any capacity for cognitive reasoning.

Chapter 5. Liar, liar, pants on fire!

"One day, when I was at the house alone—your momma had gone into town—three assholes showed up at the house armed with bowie knives, trying to rob me. They thought they had me, until they saw I had my Ruger .357 magnum in my hand. I told them to get the fuck off my land."

"What are you talking about?" I argued, looking away from the T.V.

He went on, "they came to the house and wanted to rob me, but I scared them off with my pistol."

"When was this, and why am I just now hearing about it?" I asked.

"I didn't want you or your momma to wor—"

"Wait! What? Let me get this straight. Three guys, armed with knives, came to rob you at home, and you—with pistol in hand—just let them go?"

"Well, the sheriff picked them up later." he tried to cover.

Bullshit.

This was one of many yarns my dad told me from time to time, but it was the first time he elaborated [with much more detail than I've rendered here]. So let me tell you why it's bullshit. First of all, like I said, Dad was a type A naval officer. At his peak he owned more than 300 firearms and was proficient with all of them. There is absolutely NO way that he would have had the drop on three armed robbers without dropping a hammer on at least one of them, if not all three. And there's ABSOLUTELY no way that he'd do all that and keep it to himself. He would have bragged about it for years. So I knew he was making it all up.

But that's not the important thing in the context of this scribble. What's important here is that he *believed* every word of it. To him, it had actually happened, and therein was the problem: he could no longer tell the difference between fact and fantasy.

"Hey, I got you something," he said to me.

"What's that, Dad?" I asked, my eyes still glued to the T.V.

"A school bus," he boasted proudly.

"A school bus?" I inquired, now fully focused on him. *This* I had to hear.

"Yep! A school bus. I got two of them!" he said.

"You got two school buses? For me? Uh, for what?" Now I was really curious.

"So you could do whatever you wanted with them," he said proudly, as if two school buses were going to help me complete my life's mission and save the world. I mean, he was happy.

I, for the life of me, had no clue why he happened upon two school buses. But, because I had nothing better to do at that particular moment, I pressed on. "Where did you get them?" I asked.

"Just up the road," he said.

"And how did you buy them?" I inquired, knowing full good and well he had zero ability to buy anything, inasmuch as he didn't have access to a computer, and he wouldn't have known how to use if he did. Also, he could no longer drive, and he had no idea even where his wallet was, so there was absolutely no chance of him purchasing any school buses.

"I made a phone call." Apparently, he had an answer for everything.

I have to admit, he had my mind racing a bit on why he would choose to conjure up two school buses, and then it occurred to me that I had been watching several episodes of *Tiny House Living.* On one particular episode, we watched a man finish out a school bus as a mobile home. As soon as that clicked, I knew exactly how to respond.

"Oh, Dad, that's great!" I exclaimed. "We can finish them out as two tiny homes and travel all over the country. It'll be awesome! We can go to the Grand Canyon, Yellowstone, Mt. Rushmore...," I went on and on.

He just beamed.

I could tell that he was made happy by the thought that he had done something so wonderful for his only son. He loved me and just wanted to make me happy. We talked about it for the rest of the evening: all the things we'd do, how the interior would be designed, how we would rebuild the engine (like we did with his old Camaro). We talked about where we'd go and what we'd see.

"That's awesome, Dad. Thank you so much. We'll go get them tomorrow." I finished, knowing that by "tomorrow" this would all be forgotten.

My point is this: I didn't argue with him during his delusions, some of which were death-defying; most were harmless yarns about this or that. But in either direction—happy or sad—I knew that it would be pointless to confront him for telling lies. As I said, to hear him tell them, they were real.

****

My advice to you is this: do not argue with a dementia patient. Meet them where they are [mentally] as much as you can and let them drone on. It's not going to hurt anything, and confrontation only leads to anger, arguments, and missed opportunities for some happy dialogue. That's not to say that you should let them go on and on about bad things. I did not let Dad go on too long about knife-wielding robbers; instead, I just changed the subject. I did, however, allow him to enjoy the thought of traveling around the country in two tiny houses, because it was a pleasant thing, and it made us both happy to enjoy the fantasy.

Here's the thing: living with an Alzheimer's patient is difficult and painful enough. If a fantastic story can bring a little respite to a terrible situation, I say go with it. Here are some things to be prepared for:

- Delusions of things not there – Dad would sometimes blurt out something like, "Do you see that fire hydrant?" to which he would be pointing. The trouble was, he was sitting in the living room, and the closest fire hydrant was outside and down the block! He saw insects, fire alarms, birds, animals, monsters—all from the comfort of his easy chair. Advice: If he "sees" a bug, kill it! If he sees a pretty bird, agree and say, "Yes, I see it too! Doesn't it have a pretty song?" If he sees danger, stand in its way and tell him not to worry—you got this! Don't say "it's not there," or "you're seeing things again!" Yes, your dementia patient *is* seeing things. *You* are not.

- Sinister stories – The most obvious example of a "darker" tall tale for Dad was the hold up. He did impart a few fables about shooting bad guys in his youth, or confronting nefarious demons, or participating in less-than-admirable deeds, and I have absolutely zero idea how his brain conjured them. I think it's akin to having weird bad dreams—kind of like the ones where you're naked on stage in front of thousands of people holding a bloody knife and a rubber chicken! These macabre stories clearly came from that same part of the brain. Keeping in mind that these were "real" to Dad as he told them, I just tried to redirect his mind like I did with the ice cream during night terrors. It usually worked well to ask him about what he wanted for dinner, or I would ask about his dog, "Where's Jack?" He obsessed over that dog, and the mere question about his whereabouts (even if Jack was sitting on Dad's lap) usually snapped him right out of it. The point I'm making is this: I never really thought that it was healthy to allow my father to remain in a dark state of mind—whether he was wide awake or having a nightmare. Again, by redirecting him to more pleasant things and avoiding argumentative responses, I was able to keep him relatively happy-go-lucky (most of the time).

- Other false (but happier) stories from long ago of adventures that never happened – Dad spun many a yarn about past life events, and who knows from whence they came. Fantasy? Old movies? Long-forgotten action/adventure books? Old fireside stories? I don't have the first clue and wouldn't venture a guess. The point is: let them spin. *This* is their "new normal." Just because it's fantasy to you does not diminish the reality it is to them. If you choose to argue with them, you are only hurting their feelings unnecessarily. All they really want is to feel normal, loved, and accepted. So let them talk. You never know what they are going to say, and you'll probably find that, sometimes, you'll both get a good laugh.

- On that note, try to keep your sense of humor. The night Dad called me an asshole in the mirror, I swear to God, Mom and I laughed until our ribs bled. And it was precisely because we could laugh about it that all three of us went to bed relatively happy that night. Imagine if I had puffed up and returned the insult... I had a choice. We laughed.

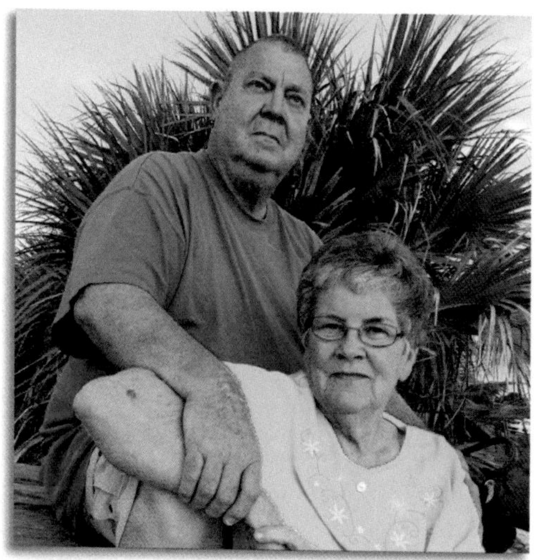

09/21/2014 – Mom & Dad on Honeymoon Island, Fl

Chapter 6. Nose dives and face plants.

One of the more dangerous aspects of dealing with a dementia patient is their loss of mobility and coordination. The first time Dad fell down was at his house on Smith Lake in Arley, Alabama, just a few months after he was diagnosed. We had no idea that this was going to become an ongoing and increasingly dangerous event for him. As his disease worsened, so, too, did the number of falls. Fortunately, I happened to be there. I was standing in their garage when I heard a big thump and a scream from my mom.

"Brian!" came the curdling yawp. "Brian!" she repeated.

Having no idea what the hubbub was all about, I bolted through the garage door through the kitchen and into the living room to find my dad face down on the living room floor and my mom in a panicked tizzy. My first thought was that he had had a heart attack, and as my mind raced through the BCLS protocols, he yelled out loud at mom.

"God damn it, woman! Shut up! I'm okay!" he griped, more embarrassed than mad, but clearly taking it out on her.

"Okay, Dad, let's calm down. Be still for a minute. Take a breath. Are you hurt?" I asked.

"I don't think so," he answered with disgust.

"Well, hold on, let's check. Are you in pain?" I started my assessment.

"No!" he said abruptly.

"Do you feel dizzy? Did you hit your head on anything?" I questioned.

"No. I'm not. I just want to get up," he said.

"Okay, here's what we're going to do. First, try to push yourself up and get your knees under you," I instructed, and he did so. "Good," I continued as I hooked the crook of my elbow under his armpit. "Now, rest on one knee and get a foot under you, and then let's try to stand up. I'll help."

He was able to get on one knee and, with my assistance, to stand up and move to his chair, where he flopped back down.

So we took a deep breath and did a quick assessment of what the fuck had just happened. He reported no dizziness, no headaches, no blackouts, no crossed shoelaces, no loose shoes, no errant squirrels in the room... *nothing* that would have caused the fall. According to him, he just lost his footing and fell down, narrowly missing a glass coffee table with his face. That would have been a disaster, so Mom and I decided right then and there to remove the table, just in case it happened again.

The second significant fall occurred after they had moved to Virginia. They had relocated so Mom would get help with his care from her brother and sister who lived in Richmond and Smithfield, respectively. She rented a two-story house less than 100 yards from her sister's home. The master bedroom was upstairs. Dad felt a bit chilled as he was preparing to come down the stairs, so he stopped at the linen closet and grabbed a blanket, then wrapped himself in it before proceeding down the 14 steps that led to a platform where 3 more steps to the right finished on the ground floor. Not paying attention to the fact that he wrapped his arms inside the blanket, which was longer than he was tall and dragging on the ground in front of him, he proceeded to step forward toward the first step. His foot, trapped within the warm cocoon he made for himself, landed on the blanket which tightened around him. His momentum now carrying his weight forward, with no way to free his arms to catch himself or brace for the fall, he fell headlong down the stairs, landing hard enough on the platform to dent the sheetrock with his head before tumbling left onto the cold tile that awaited his massive weight to finally come to rest. It was only by the grace of God that he broke no bones and didn't kill himself right there. It was truly miraculous that he didn't break his neck. Bruised a bit, but not seriously injured, he had to wait on my cousin's husband, Brien, to come over and help him off the floor.

After they moved to Florida, Mom bought a small villa in Oldsmar, in the East Lake Woodlands community. The path that led to the front door was three long steps covered in sharp slate rock. Mom and I both commented that we'd have to be really careful getting him up and down those steps. Predictably, our fears were confirmed on more than one occasion. Most of the time, I was able to catch him and keep him from falling all the way to the ground. However, he did manage to escape my grasp on two occasions. Once, before I moved in and wasn't there, he face-planted coming down the steps on the concrete sidewalk below the slate steps. That left a mark for a few days, but again, nothing serious. And once while I was there, he was walking up the steps and tripped trying to scale the first hurdle. I saw that he was falling toward the sharp edge of the slate. Realizing in an instant that I didn't have the time, nor was I in the right position to catch his fall, I heaved my shoulder with all my body weight behind it into his ribs and knocked him sideways onto the grass rather than letting him continue his fall toward the sharp, solid rock. He skinned his knee on the edging, but other than that and having the wind knocked out of him by my NFL maneuver, he was okay. It would have been much worse, I think, if he had landed on the slate. I suppose all those years of football in my youth had finally paid off.

Dad fell often; more often than I'd care to share. We were fortunate that he wasn't brittle and never broke any bones nor suffered any more than a few scrapes and bruises. As the Alzheimer's progressed, he was less and less able to render aid in our attempts to get him back up.

The last time he fell was only a few days before he went to hospice. It was bedtime, and he tripped over the edge of the carpet. He was so disoriented that he couldn't understand my instructions to help me get him back up. I couldn't move 300+ pounds of floppy dead weight by myself. He just wasn't getting it, so after an hour of wrestling with him, getting nowhere and straining my back so badly that I could barely move, we called the fire department at about 2:00 a.m. I thought it was pretty embarrassing, but the guys at East Lake Fire & Rescue, Station 56, were very gracious and understanding. They assured me that this wasn't their first rodeo with such a call and asked me to step aside.

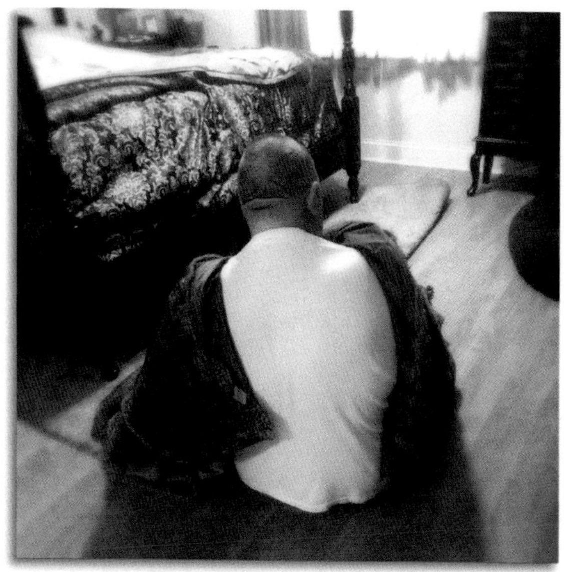

02/06/2016 – Eleven days before his death, Dad fell on his way to bed and couldn't get up. He just sat there, waiting on paramedics to arrive. It was his last fall.

Two paramedics, one on each arm, snatched him up in a jiffy! Heck, they even made it look easy. *Thanks, guys.*

****

Avoiding falls will be a high priority for your dementia patient. There are a few things you should do to prevent any falls, but inasmuch as it is highly unlikely you'll be able to stop them, there are some things you can do to make them less frequent, and/or less apt to cause serious injury. We were just plain lucky. However, we did take the following precautions:

- Remove any glass coffee tables, end tables, and any other furniture that--if fallen upon—would likely break into shards or dangerous pieces.
- Get a walker. Dad had a very high-end walker, complete with hand brakes and a built-in seat (plus it was crimson red, his favorite Alabama Crimson Tide color!). The seat was perfect. It made it possible for the walker to double as a wheelchair. That came in handy on several occasions.
- One of his physical therapists showed us how to use a "gait belt"—a long, thick, cotton belt that she wrapped around his torso to do many things: lift him up, prevent him from falling when walking, etc. There are several types of similar devices, and you can find them with a quick internet search for "Gait Belt."

- Consider a motorized lift chair. We got one for Dad, and it was one of the best decisions we ever made for him, especially as he was less and less able to lift himself up. And even when he couldn't understand the command to get up, he certainly understood it when we pushed the button to lift him out of the chair. Worked like a charm.

- We always walked very close to Dad after he started falling. As many times as he did fall, there were countless times we caught him—far more than the number of times he found the floor. Advice: if they are up, you should never be more than an arms-length away. Oh, and be prepared to act at all times.

Chapter 7. Can you just talk to me?

Dad and I had a tenuous relationship. Even during the happiest of times, I knew not to bother him with any of my real feelings. His heroes were warriors—John Wayne, Clint Eastwood, Charles Bronson—you know, The Dirty Dozen kind of guy who showed no fear, killed bears with his bare hands, plowed fields without horses, busted through brick walls with his fists, never backed down from a fight and always won, and yet could sweep a pretty woman off her feet and pat a little girl on the head and tell her everything was going to be all right just before singled-handedly fighting off a raid of murderous marauders. He was a man—a *real* man. And if ever you had any notion that you were a man—or wanted to become one—you sure as shit better walk like one if you wanted to stay on his good side.

Emotions were not allowed. I'm 57 years old as I type these words, and I can vividly remember Dad's glare as far back as when I was six and him telling me, "quit crying or I'll give you something to cry about!" And he would. He used to rebuild Chevrolet Corvairs back in the day. I don't know what his obsession was about those cars, but he loved them. He would go to junk yards and buy two or three junk Corvairs at a time, piecemeal one good one out of the lot and sell it. On one such rebuild, he was lying on his back underneath the car when he yelled for me to get him a 9/16" boxed-end wrench. I remember the term distinctly, because I had no clue what a "boxed-end wrench" even looked like. I was six! As the adrenaline coursed through my veins, the fear of impending doom swept over me. I began this torrid treasure hunt looking through his three gray Craftsman toolboxes for a wrench with a box on the end of it. And there I was... with tears in my eyes, struggling to find the right wrench when I heard that dreaded shriek, "God damn it, boy! Don't make me get out from under this car! It's right there in the second toolbox!"

A minute later, he was out from under the car, steaming mad, because I couldn't find the tool he needed. He huffed into the carport shed and continued his rant, "God damn it, Son, this isn't hard. It's right here," he barked as he fumbled through his "second" toolbox. Not there. Then he bitched and pissed and hissed and moaned and grumbled while he looked through his "first" toolbox... and then his "third." Not there, either.

"Shit!" he said, now standing erect with his six-foot frame looming above me—scared shitless and crying like a baby—looking up at him with only a singular desire to please him in my heart. "What did you do with it?" he accused, right about the time he noticed something that abruptly stopped his rant at the six-year-old crybaby quivering at his feet. And there it was ...at his eye level, on a shelf in the shed, a good two feet above my head. "God damn it!" He said, as he grabbed the wrench and started back to the underbelly of the car. "Quit your crying and get outta here," he finished with me, unapologetically. That was my dad—a gruff old fart.

I have many other stories about my youth under the macho tutelage of my John Wayne-wannabe father, but like I said in the prologue, this is not my story, and I don't want to get into it. The point I'm making is this: my father was largely unavailable for me growing up—emotionally, I mean. He never particularly wanted to know how I was doing, or how I felt, or what might be bothering me at any given time. When he barked, he expected me to jump as high as I could and pray it was high enough. No matter what successes I may have had, he was always there to point out how I could have done this or that better, or how I missed a spot. If I had cured cancer with an injection, I'm sure he'd bitch the needle was too big. Over the years, especially as an adult when his opinions became less important than those of my friends and professional peers,

I learned to tune out his little jabs, or—in the more heated moments—I'd just tell him to go fuck himself. Of course, by then I was a grown man and an ex-cop, so he knew fucking with me might cost him some teeth.

****

On a personal note: Having told you that story, I feel compelled to point out that, while my dad did have his character flaws and certainly was no saint, life with him wasn't always so insensitive and abusive. He did love us, and he absolutely provided for the family. His mother died when he was only seven, and his father—an abusive, uneducated alcoholic—married a prostitute to replace her. The result was that my dad never really learned how to show love. In his mind, the provisions of home, toys, food, and clothing were his manner of exhibiting his affection for the family. He grew up so poor he had to borrow a pair of shoes to wear to his high school graduation. He was also bounced around from family member to family member, as his father and new bride had little time to raise a pesky little boy. Even though he could be a prick and rarely displayed any outward affection for me, I still knew he loved me, so let's cut him some slack.

****

Fast forward to the fall of 2015. Dad's Sundowner's syndrome was working its magic, and I knew it was going to be "one of those nights." After wrestling with him up and down, up and down, for nearly six hours, I gave in, decided yet again to forego sleeping, and took him to the living room to watch T.V., so Mom could get some sleep. All three of us were mad; Mom and I because we couldn't sleep, and Dad because he didn't know what the fuck the fucking fuck was.

I got him situated in his chair and, with a deep drawn-out sigh of disgust, I flopped onto the love seat, reached for the remote and flipped on the tube. He was rambling about God knows what. Frankly, I didn't give a shit. I just let him ramble. I was tired, irritable, pissed, generally in a cranky mood, and I was trying to find something decent to watch at 2:00 a.m., and then Dad suddenly said something that stopped my heart cold.

"Son," he said. "Can you just talk to me?"

I looked over at him. He was looking at me with these big, tear-filled eyes, longing for some kind of connection to something, someone, anyone, me—his son. I just looked at him. Stunned for a moment, my jaw dropped open, and my mind raced through a gamut of reactions. I turned off the television and responded sympathetically, "Sure, Daddy. What would you like to talk about?"

It was at that moment that I realized how absolutely isolating the disease had become for *him.* He was no longer the gruff old fart. He was a lonely, scared, and confused human being who just needed some comfort, care, companionship, connection ...*love*. He—at that moment—needed me to simply love him.

We talked until the sun came up. What about? Absolutely everything and nothing at all. I pretended he was all there mentally, and I asked him all sorts of questions that a son might have for his father. He gave me his meandering, incoherent answers, and I just nodded and agreed, as if they all made perfect sense. To him they did.

****

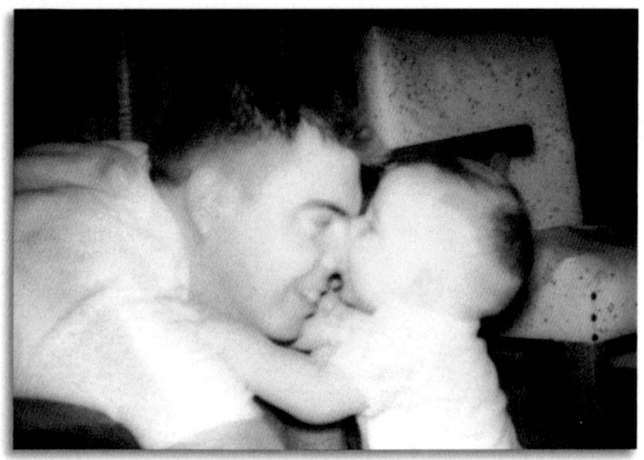

Dad and me, Fall of 1963

When you are fighting the daily fight of cleaning shit, scraping diarrhea off the walls, mopping piss, changing diapers, arguing with foul mood shifts, and restless nights, it's easy to forget that you are dealing with a human being—not just a "chore" that needs doing. Talk to them. *TALK to them.* They need love and affection, too.

From that point on, I spent time talking to Dad. I hugged him at night when I put him to bed and kissed his forehead as if he were a little boy. "Good night, Dad," I'd say with a kiss, "sweet dreams," as I would lay him down and turn off the light. *Of course, that'd only last about 5 minutes (sigh).*

Chapter 8. Get your shit together, right now!

If I were to rewrite this book in terms of chronological need, this would be Chapter 1: What should you do *first* after your loved one is diagnosed? Just to be on the safe side, I consulted a good friend of mine, Mr. Lee Carr, an elder law attorney in Florida[1], who helped me craft this list of "MUST-Do's" to ensure that you, the caregiver, and your loved one, the patient, are legally protected and retain the desired authority over patient care, treatments, final arrangements and management of the estate as the disease progresses unto death. Procrastination on getting these things done may lead to the loss of your authority over care, treatments, hospitals and extended care facilities, final arrangements, and even the final estate after death. If your loved one is declared mentally incompetent before these documents are in place, then you've lost control. Don't let that happen to you! I urgently suggest that you consult a local elder law attorney in your area and start getting your shit together, *right now*!

[1] Lee Carr II, Elder Law, Carr Law Group, PA, 111 2nd Ave., NE, Suite 1401, St. Petersburg, FL 33701

I cannot stress enough how vital it is to take these measures as soon as possible!

1. ***Durable* Power of Attorney (POA)** – Probably the single most important document to get in place as soon as possible is the *Durable* Power of Attorney. It must be "durable" in order for the "power" to remain in force after the patient is declared mentally incompetent by a doctor, and yes, that day *will* come. A standard POA yields temporary power and becomes null and void if ever the grantor is mentally incapacitated. For example: many car dealerships will have you sign a temporary POA so they can order license tags on your behalf when you buy a new car, but, if you were to have a stroke immediately after you signed that document, it would be worthless, and the dealer would no longer retain the power to act on your behalf. If you do not have this type of durable POA—especially if there are any antagonists in the family with differing opinions on care and final arrangements, etc.—the State has the authority to step in and assign an outside agent (usually a lawyer) to act as a legal guardian, who will then have absolute authority to manage all manner of care, selection of facilities,

hospice, and final arrangements (if not already governed by a will).

2. **Living Will** – A living will provides final instructions to doctors and caregivers after the patient loses consciousness and can no longer visibly respond to questions. Dad fell into a coma on a Wednesday night and remained in that state for eight days before he passed away. The instructions in his living will were to only provide comfort care (e.g., pain medications to keep him comfortable) but not any life-sustaining measures (like ventilators or food pumps, etc.). Dad did not want to live as a vegetable, and his desires to die with dignity were expressed in his living will. Without this document, either the doctor or the State would have made those decisions for him.

3. **Last Will and Testament** – It boggles my mind in this day and age at how many grown adults don't have a will. In some cases, where there is nothing to leave and no loved ones left behind, I suppose a will may be moot; however, for the rest of us, I cannot think of a more important document to have. Moreover, not only should you have one, you should also register it with your local Probate Office. The last thing you need in the aftermath of a family member's death is a probate

judge sticking their nose into your private life. It's so simple to avoid that frustration, and yet I've heard horror story after horror story of folks with significant estates who died without a will leaving plenty of survivors to fight over the decedent's assets. Personally, I think it's irresponsible not to have one. Thank God, my dad had his will in order. By the time he died, he had very little to fight over, and neither my mom nor I had even the slightest interest in fighting over what he left. Still, it was one less worry we had to deal with. For larger estates with multiple [potential] beneficiaries, a Last Will and Testament will establish how the estate is to be divvied up among the recipients. Even if there is a sole inheritor, such as a spouse, some states make it very difficult to take actions related to the leftover estate in the absence of a will. There are many things to consider: estate taxes (a.k.a. a "death tax"), property taxes, debts, business ownership (and any related licensure, taxes, or debts therefor), ex-spouses, children from previous marriages, etc., etc. All of these frustrations can be easily avoided with a well-crafted will.

4. **Social Security** – My dad was retired from the Navy, which meant he collected both social security and

military retirement pay. Dealing with both of these government agencies had its challenges. Sometimes I think government entities purposefully increase the frustration factor just to avoid actually doing the work! Nonetheless, it had to be done. I'm not going to go into a great deal of detail here on the specific requirements, because I know that one of the favorite things for government agencies to do is change the rules every year, so whatever I write today about what happened years ago may already be obsolete! That said, there are a few things I'm sure of. For starters, the Social Security Administration (SSA) will eventually require that you establish a "representative payee" for your loved one to whom the patient's social security benefits will be paid. This will require a separate bank account for that purpose. The "representative payee"—in our case, my mother—was then responsible for how my father's social security benefits were to be spent (for rent/mortgage, daily living expenses, etc.). There are some specific rules of engagement for a representative payee regarding how the money can and cannot be spent; for instance, they may frown if you use the funds for frivolous, self-serving expenditures. You are the representative for a reason; presumably to provide oversight and fiscal stewardship, not for personal gain. The SSA will provide those guidelines when the time comes.

Again, it's important to have this done before the doctor's declaration of mental incompetence. If the patient still has the ability to grant permission to his/her representative, it will alleviate the need to get doctor statements later on (which we had to do, because we didn't know about the program until after Dad was declared). Best advice is to visit your local SSA office early, obtain their instructions, and start the process. Having said that, my advice is to go sometime Tuesday through Thursday, as early in the morning as possible. It's like going to the DMV and may take a while. They always seemed to be mobbed on Mondays and Fridays.

5. **Military Retirement Account (if applicable)** – Fortunately, we could manage Dad's military retirement account through the "MyPay" portal at https://mypay.dfas.mil. Dad shared his login and password information with Mom and me, so we had no difficulty getting statements or directing deposits. For any of you who have a retired military patient and do not have the requisite login information, you can reach out for guidance to the Defense and Financial

Accounting Service at 888-332-7411 or visit the website at https://dfas.mil.

Important Note: Military retirement is paid at the beginning of the month. When a retired veteran dies during the month, after pay has been distributed, they will debit the pay account for that month's pay *regardless of the day he or she dies*. Dad died on February 17th, and the DFAS debited his account for the full month's pay relatively quickly after they were notified of the death; i.e., within a week or two. It would not have mattered if he had died on the 28th of February, we would have still lost the whole month of pay. The debit is not prorated, so be prepared for that. We weren't, and it immediately put my mother into financial duress. It sucked.

6. **Bank Accounts** – Mom and Dad always had joint accounts, so she never had any difficulties accessing money. I won't pretend to be a financial advisor, and I would never dream of telling anyone how to manage their money. However, I do know this: joint accounts made access possible without having to go through probate, so I would highly recommend that you make proper arrangements that ensure you have access to all accounts when the time comes. If you do have a

financial advisor, then I would suggest that you reach out to them, apprise them of the situation and follow their trusted guidance. If you do not have one, the elder law attorney you choose can probably guide you based on your state and local laws and in accordance with final wishes. The important thing to know is that you should make these financial arrangements sooner than later in the process—first of all, because it needs to be done before mental incompetence is declared, and secondly, because you're going to have less and less free time to deal with these necessary chores as the disease progresses.

7. **Final Arrangements** – No one likes to think about their own mortality. We didn't, and Dad certainly did not want to even discuss the matter other than to say, "Just cremate me and spread my ashes in Smith Lake with Tracy." He was referring to my sister who was cremated and spread there after she was murdered in 1999. Prior to her death, he just wanted to be buried in a plain pine box, and God forbid he have any kind of formal funeral! No, no, no... that would not do!

   Dad had some pretty firm opinions about how his final arrangements were to be made, but never took a moment's time planning for them. That would be on me. In fact, whenever I tried to get him to take any sort of action toward planning arrangements, he would only scoff, "That's not my problem, Son. That's YOUR problem!" And right he was. *Marvelous.*

This is what I know to be absolutely certain about the funeral industry: most of them are nothing more than thieves, and as far as I'm concerned, they can kiss my ass. After Dad was admitted to hospice, the nurse handed me a list of all the local funeral homes, complete with all the necessary contact information (addresses, phone numbers, emails, etc.). During the week he lay dying, I started down the list and started asking about the cost of cremation. The prices varied from $1,700 to $7,500. I was perplexed; why, on God's green earth, was it so expensive to cremate someone in Florida, and why was there such variance in cost from one funeral home to the next? *What... did they have varying degrees of being burnt to ashes?* Was one fire *better* than another? I happened to call the crematory under the name "Abbey Affordable Crematory" and found out why. One word: greed.

Abbey Affordable was the very same crematory that most of the local funeral homes were using, and they charged the general public the exact same amount that they charged a funeral home – $695. That's right, 695 was their number, plus a bit more for urns or legal copies of death certificates (which you will need, by the way). Long story, short... I was all in for less than $900. That included two tiny urns—one each for mom and me—and ten death certificates (five each of both long and short forms).

Here's the thing: I'm not in any way, shape, or form going to tell you what kind of funeral you should have for yourself or for your loved one. What I *am* going to say is that it's best to plan ahead, whether you want the cheapest, simplest thing you can find or a five million-dollar mausoleum with a marching band and a parade of hula girls. Do your shopping *before* you die. The average cost of a simple, plain funeral these days is about $25k, and nothing makes a funeral director salivate more than an "at-need" client who walks in the door grieving over a fresh death. They love playing on those emotions and make no mistake—they're going to try to fuck you. ...Just sayin'

So, shop while you are thinking relatively clearly. And shop around!

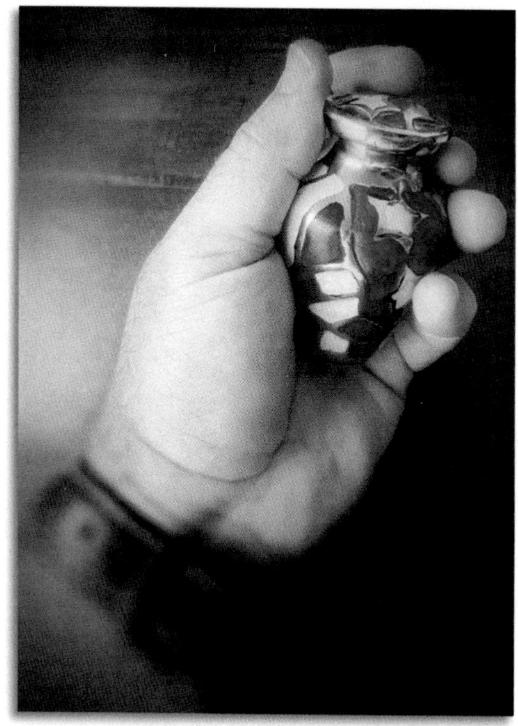

Dad's Tiny Keepsake Urn

Chapter 9. Salvation.

The matter of one's faith is very personal, so much so that I struggled with the notion of omitting this chapter altogether. Ultimately, I decided to keep it for a few reasons. First of all, I do believe that God is worthy of praise, and I'd like to give credit where credit is due. I would feel uncomfortably remiss if I had simply left Him out.

Secondly, I wanted to end my work on a positive note for reasons that will be readily apparent in the next chapter. I saved this chapter as the last I would actually write to remind myself that I will indeed see my daddy again. *This* is what made the whole journey worth the pain, suffering, exhaustion, tears, and effort to get here. *This* makes my heart smile. I hope it makes yours smile, too.

****

Dad was more of an agnostic than an atheist. He certainly was not spiritual. He claimed to have read the Bible through and through twice, only then to lay it down and proclaim that it was all bullshit. When pressed, he would tell you that he believed there was "something out there" greater than the sum of man's understanding and that we [humans] had been planted on this planet by some other intelligent lifeform eons ago. He never gave it much more thought, other than to mock anyone of faith as merely sheep being fleeced for their money. He was less than enthused when I accepted the Lord and became a Christian on Father's Day, June 18th, 1995.

I had been invited to church by the pastor, Rick Johnson, whose sons I had coached with my own in little league baseball. I went reluctantly, feeling obligated to a man who had helped so much with the team during the course of the season. I'll never forget the sermon he preached that Sunday at Friendship Baptist Church (formerly Triana Village Baptist) in Huntsville. The title was "The Godly Man vs. the Worldly Man," and he compared and contrasted the lives of the former vs. the latter. Every time he described the worldly man, I knew that was me, and every time he described the Godly man, I knew it wasn't. By the time he wrapped up the sermon, my palms were wet with sweat, and my legs where shaking. I stumbled down the aisle along the right side of the church to get to the altar at the end of the service, and looking up at Rick, all I could muster was, "Can you help me?"

He did that by sharing with me some key verses in the Bible that I would later learn are called, "The Roman

Road;" that is, verses that illustrate succinctly the Gospel of Christ in such a manner that even the unlearned can understand its meaning. He led me in the Sinner's Prayer and the Spirit immediately fell upon me like a warm blanket in a cold winter storm. It literally changed my life.

Before I go much further, I acknowledge right here and now that I am a very poor example of a Christian. I cuss like the son of a sailor and ex-cop that I am. I no longer attend church regularly. I drink from time to time, and I smoke cigars. I am, by far, not what you would expect to draw if asked to paint a picture of a perfect Christian. By definition, I am still a sinner. Still, the whole point of Christianity is God's grace manifested in His forgiveness for wayward souls like mine. The only requirement—per the Gospel—is that I acknowledge my sins and the fact that Christ died on the cross for them in my stead, and finally to ask for the grace of God's forgiveness, which I have done. So, like it or not, yes, I am a Christian.

Getting my father to accept the Lord would be a different story. Of course, as most new Christians do, I tried to explain to him why I had made my decision and why I wanted him to do likewise.

****

Quick note here for the non-believers who don't understand this particular aspect of Christianity; I mean the part about why we want everybody else to become Christians, too. For a Christian to express their faith, it's not meant to be an insult or a judgment. It's more like a "rescue" of sorts. If you saw someone standing in the middle of the street, and a bus was barreling down at them, wouldn't you say something? Wouldn't you at least yell at them to get out of the way? Or run out and push them out of the street? You see, in our hearts, we believe that not accepting Christ is the *only* unforgivable sin. It's akin to turning your back on God's gift—i.e., Jesus, his "only begotten Son"—and subsequently, Heaven. There's nothing you can do to earn it, either. Being a "good person" doesn't cut it; I mean how good do you have to be, *exactly*? How would you *know* you're good enough? It's a gift, given by grace, through faith. Period. That is the *quintessential essence of God's grace,* i.e., that you *can't* earn it. You *must* ask for it.

****

So, yes, I very much wanted my father to accept Christ and secure his place in Heaven. I bought him a Bible that Christmas with his name embossed on it and highlighted a passage in Proverbs which reads:

> *[1]Hear, ye children, the instruction of a father, and attend to know understanding.*
> *[2]For I give you good doctrine, forsake ye not my law.*
> *[3]For I was my father's son, tender and only beloved in the sight of my mother.*
> *[4]He taught me also, and said unto me, Let thine heart retain my words: keep my commandments, and live.*
> *~Proverbs 4:1-4, KJV*

He accepted the gift, read the passage, and put it down without saying a word. I'm sure he thought I'd snapped a twig and silently hoped one day I would just come to my senses and outgrow this "phase" and my faith would pass. I would spend the next 20 years praying for my dad to "see the light."

****

"I like that song," Dad said aloud.

I had my iPhone wired into my car's sound system and *Amazing Grace*, sung by Lari White on the album *Amazing Grace: A Country Salute to Gospel,* had just spun up randomly. "I do, too," said my mom.

"Really?" I asked my dad, incredulous that he would even acknowledge a gospel song out of the myriad random songs in my 4,200+ library that included everything from rock, country, jazz, blues, classical, bluegrass, folk, ...whatever.

"Yes," he reconfirmed, "I like it a lot."

Hmmm... I thought. I reached for the phone, switched it from random play to the album. *Let's see about that.*

The next song in line was *Peace in the Valley*, sung by John Anderson. "How about that one?" I asked my dad.

"Yes, it's beautiful," he continued. "I really like this. I've never heard it before."

We were just out shopping and generally driving around to break the monotony of staying at the house. Mom wanted to go to a few stores and specifically wanted to stop at Michael's on US Highway 19 in Palm Harbor. I pulled in the parking lot and found a space to bring my Lincoln MKZ to rest.

"Coming in?" Mom queried, as she opened the door to get out of the car.

"Not this time, Mom. You go ahead," I answered. *I've got something else to do.*

Just as when I received the Lord in 1995, I suddenly felt that familiar, warm blanket wrap around my shoulders. *Now! Now, is the time. It's now or never.* As Mom disappeared into Michaels, I turned my attention to my father in the seat next to me.

"Dad," I asked, "I'm curious. Have you even given any more thought about Heaven? Or where you might go after you die?"

"You know I think that's all bullshit," he objected. "I've led a good life."

"Yes," I agreed, "but has it been good enough? I mean, how do you *know*?"

"I don't," he said, now looking right at me.

"Do you believe you have always been good? I mean, have you not made mistakes? Maybe even done some wrong things that you regret?"

"I'm not perfect. Don't claim to be," he acknowledged.

"The last time we talked about this, you didn't want to hear it. Do you mind if I show you some things in the Bible?" I pressed.

His head dropped as he pondered the question. He looked back up with a very serious expression. I had no idea what was going through his mind, but I could tell that something was different. I guess it really dawned on him that he was getting closer to the end. He quietly nodded and said, "Let's hear it."

My heart leapt! I could barely believe that this was happening. He *wanted* to hear it. I opened the KJV Bible app on my phone, quickly found Romans 3:10 and 3:23:

3:10 As it is written, there is none righteous, no not one.
3:23 For all have sinned and fallen short of the glory of God.

"This means exactly what you just said about yourself, Dad. No one is perfect in the sight of God. All of us are sinners. Do you understand?" I asked.

"Yes," he said in a whisper.

Then came Romans 5:12 and 6:23:

5:12 Wherefore, as by one man sin entered into this world, and death by sin; and so death passed upon all men, for that all have sinned.
6:23 For the wage of sin is death; but the gift of God is eternal life through Jesus Christ our Lord.

"This means that a price must be paid for our sins. Do you know what that is, Dad?" I asked, watching carefully to make sure he understood.

"Death," he said without emotion.

"That's right, Dad—death. But the good news is the gift of God is *eternal* life," I continued, "Do you understand what that means?"

"Heaven," he said, now looking up at me as if he knew something unexpected was next.

"Right! Dad, that's right!" I riffled to John 3:16:

> *For God so loved the world, that he gave his only begotten Son, that whosoever believeth in him should not perish but have everlasting life.*

And then I read the final verse, Romans 10:9:

> *That if thou shalt confess with thy mouth the Lord Jesus, And shall believe in thine heart that God hath raised him from the dead, thou shalt be saved.*

"You see, Dad, all we have to do to get into Heaven is acknowledge that we are sinners and accept that Christ paid the price of death *for our sins* by dying on the cross *for us*. That's it. Nothing else." I explained and then asked, "Do *you* want to do that now, Dad? All we have to do is pray. We can do it together..." I held my breath.

He nodded and with a whisper simply said, "Yes."

Placing my hand on his shoulder, we bowed our heads together, and I led him through the Sinner's Prayer that goes something like this:

> Dear Lord, I come to You now, a humble sinner, to acknowledge that I have sinned before You. I accept that You sent your Son, Jesus, to pay the price for my sins, and I ask for your grace and forgiveness. I'm asking You now to come into my heart, Lord, and help me find my place in Yours. Amen.

When we finished, he looked up with an ear-to-ear grin I'll never forget.

****

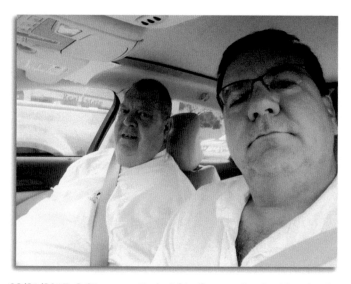

08/31/2015, 2:01 p.m. – Dad, right after praying for his salvation.

Now I know what you're thinking: the man had Alzheimer's, for crying out loud! How could he possibly be lucid enough to make such a decision? Well, all I have to offer you is my faith and this Bible passage about how to approach God for salvation, that is with the mind of a child. Mark 10:14-15:

[14]But when Jesus saw it, he was much displeased, and said unto them, Suffer the little children to come unto me, and forbid them not: for of such is the kingdom of God.

[15]Verily I say unto you, Whosoever shall not receive the kingdom of God as a little child, he shall not enter therein.

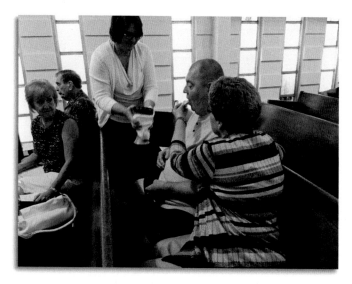

Dad receives communion for the first (and last) time at Sylvan Abbey Methodist Church in Clearwater, FL.

Stripped of his machismo, I'm pretty sure dad had the mind of a child when he prayed that day, and he definitely gave the right answers when asked, so... on this one... I'll just have to it take on faith that maybe, *just maybe,* God might have had a bigger reason for Dad's illness. I guess I'll find out when I get to Heaven. Will you?

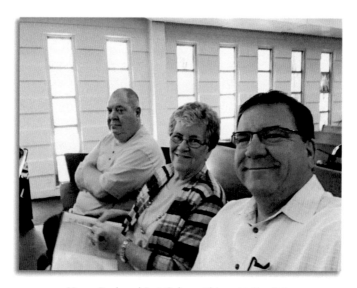

Mom, Dad and I at Sylvan Abbey Methodist
after communion.

Chapter 10. This is the end.

The most disturbing part of Alzheimer's is the long, painful, degenerative road to the end. When you're going through it, it's hard to pick out the milestones, and even harder to see the light at the end of the tunnel. In my dad's final days, he slept more than he was awake, he ate less food, drank less fluid, became more and more lethargic, and often complained that he didn't feel well. When asked to describe how he felt, he could only say that he felt "funny," and on one ominous day he actually said, "I feel like I'm dying." He was dead less than two weeks after that.

In December of 2015, there were two tragedies unfolding in our lives. My dad's disease was taking its toll, and my aunt Weezie—my mom's only sister—was dying of cancer in Virginia. We had no way of knowing that my dad and my aunt would die eight days apart on the 17th and 25th of February, respectively, but we did know that Christmas '15 was the last that either of them would celebrate. It was the elephant in the room the week before Christmas when I overheard my mom talking to her sister on the phone. Both of them were in tears and lamenting that they couldn't be together this one last time. She hung up and bawled. That's all I could take.

"Get packed," I announced. "We're going."

"What, where?" Mom asked.

"We're going to Virginia. You are going to see your sister this Christmas. I'm not arguing about it. We're going. If we leave now, we can be there by sun-up."

With that, we packed our bags, settled Dad in the shotgun seat, scooped up the dogs, and hit the road.

Normally, it's about a 14-hour drive from Clearwater to Smithfield. Our luck wasn't quite so good. It rained the whole time, and not just a gentle shower either—it was pouring to beat the band. That, plus all the other holiday travelers on the road (driving like complete idiots, I might add) resulted in a 19-hour ordeal that—until the ride home—was the absolute worst road trip I had ever driven.

Driving through the night is my preferred way to take long road trips, because there's usually less traffic and even fewer distractions. *Usually* is the operative word. As the night progressed, my dad's Sundowner's was kicking into high gear. He couldn't comprehend why we were in the car for so long, and like a child in the way-far-back seat of a family station wagon, he interrupted the trip often with "are we there yet?" questions, and "I gotta go pee!" exclamations! It was grueling, but we finally got there sometime before noon the next day, just in time for Dad to pass out and sleep, perched on a recliner in my aunt's living room. I took the opportunity to escape to a hotel room.

I was completely exhausted. I had to find a bed. Fast. Fortunately, I had about a bazillion frequent-user points at the Hampton Inn from my previous job when I had travelled so often, and my stay was very cheap. I remember thinking, as I stretched across the bed, how nice it was not to have to take care of Dad for the next few hours. It was a short respite.

Mom and Weezie were elated in a bittersweet sort of way. They got to spend their last Christmas together. Mom stayed with her sister. Dad and I stayed at the hotel, which meant that I was not getting any sleep at all. His Sundowner's always seemed more intense because we were in a strange place that he didn't recognize and felt insecure. I'd put him to bed and 15 minutes later, he'd be yelling at me for some unknown torment he was suffering—be it some bad guys trying to get him, demons on the loose, dogs in the kitchen, ducks in the bathtub ...or whatever.

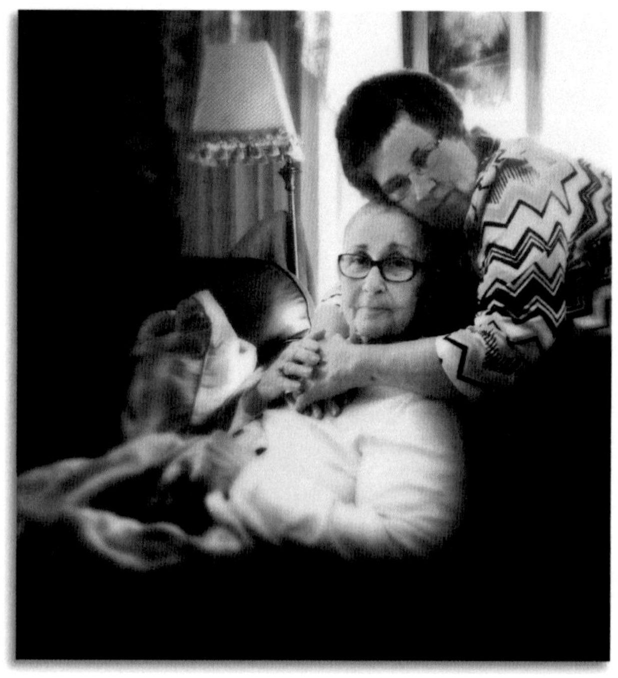

Christmas Day, 2015 – Mom with her sister
Louise "Weezie" Whittkamp
05/23/1942 – 02/25/2016

After spending Christmas Day with extended family at my cousins' house, complete with in-laws, bouncing kids, barking dogs, loud televisions, family arguments, tears, laughter, and reminiscences of better times, it was finally time to return to the hotel and prepare for the trip home the next day. This time, I planned to leave in the morning and drive during daylight hours, erroneously thinking Dad would handle the trip south better than he did the ride north. Yeah... so much for that.

Little did any of us know that we had just embarked on a 22-hour marathon of torrential downpours, clogged interstates, crawling traffic, bad drivers, scary night-road delusions, and cheap fast food. It was absolutely awful and remains to this day the worst road trip I've ever taken.

We were up and at 'em around 7:00 a.m.; all packed, loaded, and tearfully heading south by 9:00 after saying our last in-person goodbyes to my aunt. By the time we got to I-95 just northwest of Emporia, we were completely aware that we were in for a long and uncomfortable ride. It was raining cats and dogs, and the overflowing holiday traffic was already moving at a snail's pace. We were in a Honda Accord, which is a nice car for a daily driver, but... stuff a 300-pound, demented man in the front passenger seat, his brokenhearted, crying wife in the back with three dogs, and a pissed off ex-cop in the driver's chair... well, let's just say it was far less than "perfect" for this particular trip.

And there we were: meandering south and trying to cope. Again, we stopped as frequently as needed for food, pee breaks, or those wonderful "I gotta go shit!" announcements of Dad's. After nine grueling hours, we still had not crossed the South Carolina/Georgia line, and traffic was mostly at a dead stop. It was time for a command decision: get off this fucking interstate! Unfortunately, I made that decision while in the straits of I-95, somewhere south of Lake Marion in the middle of friggin' nowhere, and it took two more hours to reach Savannah, where we finally got off 95 and plotted another pathway home. That turned out to be the best decision of the trip. The backroads were relatively empty, but it still took nearly three hours to get to Jacksonville. It was well after dark by then, and we skirted through the rain around Jacksonville right about the time I had hoped to be pulling into our driveway, which was still another 6-7 hours away on wet, mostly unlit backroads. It was around 2:00 a.m. when we passed through Gainesville and it was pitch black, but the rain had finally subsided. Dad had been agitated the whole trip. He hadn't fared well on the trip up or the stay in a strange hotel, and now he was all out of sorts with fear. He boiled over at about 2:30 a.m. and blurted loudly, "Stop! Stop! We need to call the police!"

"Why do we need to do that, Dad?" I asked impatiently.

"We're lost!" he said, with a petrified look like a small child lost alone in a dark forest, staring through the front window at the unlit black path in front of us.

Given my own level of discomfort, I wasn't really in the mood for this shit, but I managed to respond with some restraint. Sensing his extreme fear, I took a breath, lowered my voice, and with a calm, hypnotic, fatherly tone, I sighed, "No, Dad, we are not lost. I know exactly where we are, and everything is going to be okay." Reaching out to rub his shoulder, I continued, "Tell ya' what... lay your head on your pillow and try to get some sleep. By the time you wake up, we'll be home, and you'll be sitting in your chair watching T.V.." Then the strangest thing happened. He laid his head down and went right to sleep.

The rest of the trip was relatively uneventful as we eventually reached US Highway 19 South on the west coast of Florida, where we once again found illuminated streetlights and ultimately found home just before 7:00 a.m.. The sun was up. Dad was wide awake.

There were two significant events in January of 2016: The Alabama Crimson Tide won their 16th National Championship to cap their 2015 season, and my daddy turned 74. He didn't realize either of them even occurred, which, under normal circumstances, would have been very big days for him. He loved Alabama. I remember the day they won their 15th National title in 2012, and he cried like a baby because he thought that would be the last one he'd ever see. For all intents and purposes, he was right. All he knew of the Tide when they won again on January 11, 2016, was that the "red team" was on T.V.

By his birthday on the 24th, he could barely comprehend that the T.V. was even on. He mostly just sat in his chair and stared into oblivion with a thousand-yard gaze. That was when he was awake, which was less and less. My dad was crossing over the "knee-bend"—that part of the curve where his degradation was changing from a gentle slope downward into a freefall. He was getting so much worse.

We called hospice.

They were wonderful. They assigned a caregiver who came three times a week to bathe and dress my dad. I was relieved that I didn't have to do it anymore. Over the next few days after his birthday, his lethargy grew, and his appetite lessened. He spoke less but seemed to smile more when one of us would walk in the room; kind of like a puppy that wags its tail when it sees another dog. He would attempt conversation but lose his train of thought before he could get two words out of his mouth and drift back into oblivion on his recliner.

On Monday, February 8th, he was writhing restlessly in his chair. "What's wrong, Daddy?" I asked, concerned.

"I don't feel good," he answered.

"What's wrong?" I inquired again.

"I dunno... it just hurts," he said with bent look on his face.

I walked over to his chair and stood close to him. I felt his forehead for a fever and pressed, "Where does it hurt?"

"I dunno," he muttered.

"Does your stomach hurt?" I asked.

"No," came the response.

"Does your head hurt?" I probed.

"No," he answered, looking up at me.

"Well, Dad, I can't help you if I don't know what's wrong. Try to explain it to me," I queried one more time.

Then he looked up at me with the oddest look—almost as if he was completely coherent at that moment—and all he said was, "It feels like I'm dying."

Being the dumbass I am, I scoffed it off and retorted, "You ain't dyin' yet, old man. Shit. You'll probably outlive us all."

The hospice orderly came Wednesday morning, February 10th, to bathe him and had a harder time than usual getting Dad in the shower. When he was finally done, he called the nurse and reported Dad's decreased mobility. Later that day she came to the house to assess Dad's condition and she, too, was alarmed. Mom and I hadn't been sleeping because the Sundowner's was at full volume, so the nurse suggested we admit him into the hospice facility to "see if we can get control of his sleeping pattern." Sure thing, we were all for that, so she called an ambulance and they took him to his bed at Suncoast Hospice on Tampa Road in Palm Harbor.

Mom and I arrived soon after and sat with him for a while, at least until the meds they gave him kicked in, and he drifted off to sleep. We went to dinner and then home, mildly excited about the prospect of getting a good, uninterrupted night's sleep. The next morning, we got up and took our time. There was no rush. We slept in a bit; whipped up a slow breakfast and got ready to go. We arrived around 9:30-10:00. Neither one of us was prepared for what we saw next.

Dad was in a coma. A fucking coma! *What the fuck?!*

"Nurse!" I bellowed. She popped in the room to find my ire.

"What did you give him? Why is he out like this? What are his meds?" I started.

"We haven't given him anything other than the morphine we gave him last night to help him sleep. This is "him" now," she explained.

"Wait. What the f—" I started to bark.

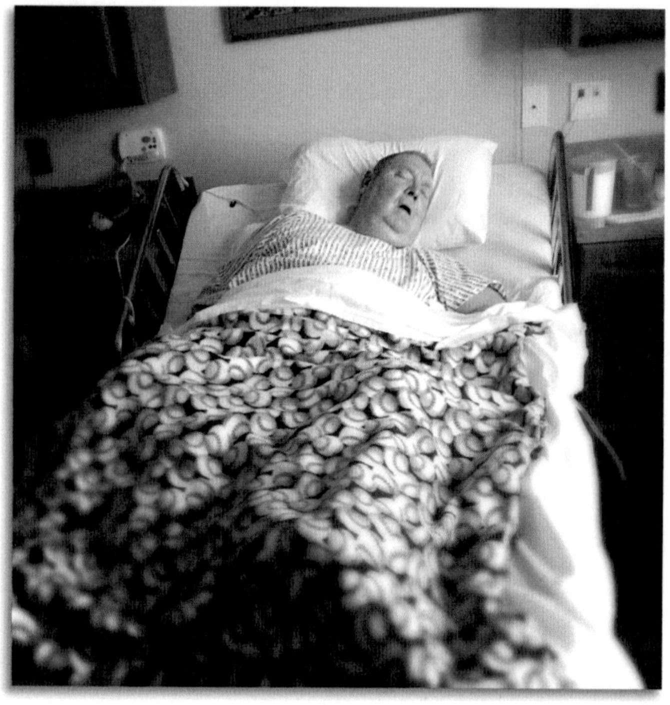

02/12/2016 – Comatose. Waiting for the inevitable.

She quickly interrupted and asked me to step outside the room before she continued, "I don't like talking in the patient's room. On some level they can hear us, and I don't want to upset your father. But you need to know this *is* his condition. He has started the dying process. He's not going home. He's not going to wake up. Do you understand?" she finished abruptly.

Her words hung in the air like a bad odor as I took a moment to absorb their meaning. "Okay," I said, trying not to choke up, "let's see what he does with no medication. Please stop all meds for 24 hours. If there's no change tomorrow, we'll keep him comfortable."

"Okay," she said calmly, placing her hand on my shoulder, knowing I had understood the full weight of her message.

24 hours later... no change. *God damn it.*

For the next week, we basically just existed one day to the next, waiting for the inevitable. Sometime around then, we also learned that Aunt Weezie was rapidly succumbing to her cancer and she, too, was moving into a hospice bed. Day in, day out... just a hazy blur, waiting and waiting.

I had signed up as a chemistry and algebra tutor on Wyzant and had one appointment for Wednesday, February 17th, at 6:00 p.m. It was a welcome break from the "death watch." I went to my appointment, but had a really uneasy feeling...

As I watched a young high-schooler trudge through the chemistry question I made up for her—calculating the moles of propellant needed to hurl a 100,000 metric ton rocket ship to the moon or something like that—my mind drifted and my anxiety level increased. I watched the clock and as soon as the minute hand crossed 7:00 p.m. I was racing back to my dad's bed. I got there around 7:30. Mom was sitting on a chair next to his bed. She stood up with a worried look on her face when I walked in and told me he was having trouble breathing. I turned my attention to him and noticed that he was indeed struggling, his chest heaving big breaths, up and down, with long breaks between them. At 8:05 he started the death rattle—starting with a big noisy breath and then almost a moan to let it out. Then another and another. Mom was in the hall just outside the room on the phone.

"Mom," I yelled for her, "this is it! Get the nurse!"

She burst into the room and gasped, "Oh, no. What do we do?"

"It's okay, Mom. Get the nurse," I said more calmly as I looked over at my dad. Mom stepped out and returned with the nurse, who placed her stethoscope on his heaving chest. She just nodded and said, "It won't be long now," and then she left.

Mom stood crying next to my dad and held his right hand. I held his left, now sitting in the chair beside his bed. His eyes opened and oddly teared up. He was looking right at me—struggling hard for every breath. He seemed to want to talk but couldn't.

"It's okay," I told him, looking into his boyish, scared eyes, "It's okay." I stroked his forehead and calmed him down. "It's okay, Daddy. You can go now. It's been a good run. You've been a good man and a good daddy. I love you. I'll see you soon. It's okay," I reassured.

He suddenly sucked in a huge breath and let it all out. Nothing...

With *Beulah Land* playing in the background on my iPhone, his eyes locked with mine, he inhaled another heaving breath. They were so far apart now that each seemed to be brand new. His lungs purged their last time, and I watched the life fade from his eyes. I glanced at the clock. It was 8:22 p.m. He was gone.

Phone calls were made. Tears were shed. And they asked us to step out while they prepped him for the funeral home, meaning they removed his catheter and IV and then cleaned him up a bit. When they opened the door for us, we had one more surprise waiting. They had draped his body with an American flag because he had been a US Navy veteran. Mom burst into tears again. We waited until the funeral home came for his body, and then we went home.

We got there around 10:00 and just sat on the love seat, side by side in that quiet house—no Sundowner's, no assholes in the mirror, no shit to clean, no diapers to change, no sound at all—just staring at a blank, black, silent television screen. Mom reached over the console between us and held my hand. We sat there indefinitely and never said a word. We didn't have to…

It had all been said.

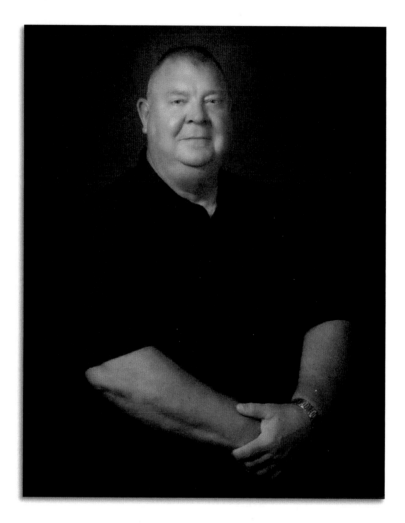

Ralph L. Morris

01/24/1942 – 02/17/2016

My Fathers Chair

This is my father's chair.
Oh, it's not his first,
But it is his just the same.
He always had "his" chair,
And through the years,
He wore it like his name.

He protected it,
Like a king would a throne.
You could sit there, if you dared.
Only when he wasn't home.

There he'd sit and watch T.V.
And yell at 'Bama games.
He'd nap and snore all reclined
And ease his daily pains.

He earned this treasured seat
Putting up with my wayward years.
He'd bark his orders and mutter advice
And sometimes shed his tears.

It's empty now, and he's not home.
He's on the other side.
The house is quiet, the chair is still,
And this pain will ne'er subside.

I stare at it and often think...
I'd like to sit there, too.
But then I fear, he's always here
And I never do.

~~~~~ * ~~~~~

Father's Day, June 18, 2016
~~~~~

Help

Accompanying this book is our website at

http://www.wipeyourdadsass.com

There you will find online resources and links to organizations that may help your personal journey with your dementia patient. You will also find many of the needed supplies mentioned in this book required for the dementia bag (gloves, KY Jelly, perineal wash, diapers, etc.), as well as some other items that may be helpful for motility and transitioning around the house.

You can also reach out to directly through our "Contact" page.

Here is our Official Facebook page where we post dementia-related stories, news:

https://www.facebook.com/howtowipeyourdadsass/

And here is our Official Facebook Group where caregivers can share and help each other cope with the day-to-day grind and issues related to dementia care:

https://www.facebook.com/groups/howtowipeyourdadsass/

Made in the USA
Las Vegas, NV
01 September 2021

29377785R00076